WHY CAN'T I REMEMBER?

REVERSING NORMAL MEMORY LOSS

WHY CAN'T I REMEMBER?

REVERSING NORMAL MEMORY LOSS

Pavel Yutsis, MD
Lynda Toth, PhD

AVERY PUBLISHING GROUP

Garden City Park • New York

The therapeutic procedures in this book are based on the training, personal experiences, and research of the authors. Because each person and situation are unique, the authors and publisher urge the reader to check with a qualified health professional before using any procedure where there is any question to appropriateness.

The publisher does not advocate the use of any particular health treatment, but believes the information presented in this book should be available to the public. Because there is always some risk involved, the author and publisher are not responsible for any adverse effects or consequences resulting from the use of any of the suggestions, preparations, or procedures described in this book. Please do not use the book if you are unwilling to assume the risk. Feel free to consult with a physician or other qualified health professional. It is a sign of wisdom, not cowardice, to seek a second or third opinion.

Cover Designer: Doug Brooks
In-House Editor: Marie Caratozzolo
Typesetter: Gary A. Rosenberg
Printer: Paragon Press, Honesdale, PA

Avery Publishing Group
120 Old Broadway
Garden City Park, NY 11040
1-800-548-5757
www.averypublishing.com

Library of Congress Cataloging-in-Publication Data

Yutsis, Pavel.
    Why can't I remember? : reversing normal memory loss / by Pavel Yutsis
and Lynda Toth.
        p.   cm.
    Includes bibliographical references.
    ISBN 0-89529-841-4
    1. Memory disorders—Popular works. I. Toth, Lynda. II. Title.
RC394.M46Y88   1999   FEB 03 2000
616.8'4—dc21   98-54421
                                                CIP

3 9082 07701 5504

Printed in the United States of America

10 9 8 7 6 5 4 3 2 1

Contents

Acknowledgments

First and foremost, I would like to thank my coauthor, Dr. Lynda Toth, for her extraordinary contribution in making this book a valuable learning source. I would also like to thank the "A-team" of Avery Publishing Group—publisher Rudy Shur and project editor Marie Caratozzolo—for their invaluable input in making *Why Can't I Remember?* such an excellent book. I will always be indebted to my "compatriots"—the complementary physicians at the Foundation for the Advancement of Innovative Medicine (FAIM), the American College for Advancement in Medicine (ACAM), and the American Academy of Environmental Medicine (AAEM)—for sharing their knowledge and love of alternative medicine. And finally, a special thank you to my lovely wife, Lilia, and my wonderful children, Max and Francine, for their love, support, and encouragement, without which this book wouldn't be possible.

Pavel Yutsis, MD

A book is the result of a collaborative effort. Many thanks to Dr. Pavel Yutsis for inviting me to be his partner in this project. Sincere regards to project editor Marie Caratozzolo for her insight and in-depth attention to the manuscript, and to publisher Rudy Shur, who was invaluable as a mentor and guiding light. Sincere appreciation is extended to Arnold Scheibel, MD, for inviting me to take his neuro-anatomy class within the UCLA School of Medicine. And profound respect goes to my parents for having the courage to allow a six-year-old to have a chemistry lab in the basement.

Lynda Toth, PhD

Introduction

"He has half the deed done, who has made a beginning."

—Horace

"Life just isn't what it used to be, Doctor Yutsis. I miss important deadlines because I don't remember to look at my organizer. Phone numbers? I have to hear them three times before I can get them straight. Why, I even forgot to meet my wife for lunch last week. I'm worried. What am I going to do?"

You may think this person is neurotic, immature, or very old. Actually, Michael is a serious-minded, responsible family man who, at forty-one, works as a systems analyst for a top company in Texas. Or take Cheryl, a pregnant, twenty-six-year-old Manhattan bookkeeper, who's having memory lapses for the first time in her life and complains she keeps losing her car keys. Then, there's thirty-three-year-old Enrique, the owner of a successful Mexican restaurant in Sacramento, who's having trouble getting phone numbers straight the third time around.

Such stories among young and middle-aged people are more common than you may think. Yet, for successful functioning in a high-tech society driven by "the competitive edge," what can be more important than a good memory? Will the people we've mentioned above have what it takes during the "full court press" of life? Can they succeed in their careers despite their memory problems?

As a clinician, I can say in all honesty that such patients are typical of a growing number of men and women in the prime of their lives who have problems remembering important details. Oftentimes, such people panic and wrongly assume their inability to remember key moments is a sign of Alzheimer's disease. And why wouldn't such patients become alarmed when statistics show that 4 million people in the United States suffer from this degenerative type of memory loss?

A closer look, however, at the Alzheimer's Association facts and figures show that nearly half of those with this serious form of dementia are over the age of eighty-five. And considering that the U.S. population is now around 271 million, Alzheimer's disease strikes only about 1.5 percent of the men and women living in this country.

Still, loss of memory is a growing concern among young and middle-aged people. So when people under age sixty-five come to my office in a cloak of secrecy, look over their shoulder, and then grimly announce they have Alzheimer's disease, I want to chuckle. But, of course, I don't. These deeply worried men and women have come to me for help and need my understanding and professional help.

My first course of action in such cases is to provide some straight facts about a more general kind of treatable memory loss that is not related to Alzheimer's disease. Once patients understand there are many other reasons why they may be having trouble remembering key details in their lives, productive memory treatment can begin.

In most situations, memory loss in middle-aged people is connected to certain life patterns in the twentieth century that expose the human brain to various kinds of chemical, biological, and/or emotional stressors. Nutritional deficiencies, free radical damage, heavy metal toxicity in the body, or sensory overload at work, at home, or at social gatherings are only some of the suspected memory robbers we will discuss in this book.

Modern life puts the human body under constant attack in a way that prior generations have never experienced. The Industrial Revolution in the late 1700s may have opened a Pandora's box of threats and dangers to the twentieth century and beyond. Scientists and doctors only now are starting to ask the kinds of questions that generate potential answers to some important questions concerning brain health.

For instance, certain biochemical reactions triggered by amino acids directly impact the brain and determine how the brain processes information. So, how do serious amino acid deficiencies harm the processing of nerve messages in the brain? Are memory cells destroyed by such shortages?

Women often suffer from decreased memory function during menopause, when estrogen levels are off balance. Since pesticides have been found in recent times to be "read" by the body as estrogen, do they also cause hormonal imbalances that could lessen memory abilities in women who are too young for this transitional period of life? Could such pesticide buildup also be affecting the memory ability of men?

Also, it's no secret that Alzheimer patients have been found to have high amounts of aluminum in their brains. Could other heavy metals be compromising human memory by destroying delicate brain tissue needed for the neurotransmission of electrical impulses? Many doctors worry, as I do, that such toxicity in key brain areas may have a negative impact on the brain's nerve signals. If this is true, memory is likely to be the first thing affected among those under toxic assault.

On top of these memory-related questions, a growing number of dentists are concerned over the possibility that the mercury in silver amalgam fillings may break down in such a way as to spread mercury through bone matter and into message processing areas of the brain. Could such mercury exposure also be a factor in memory loss in thirty-, forty-, or fifty-year-old people?

Just about anything connected to an electrical circuit radiates an electromagnetic field while it operates, creating low-frequency radiation. This means that bedside clock radios may be doing more than waking us up in the morning. A large population study sponsored by the Swedish government in the 1980s found that electromagnetic force fields can affect cellular tissue, causing negative impact on the immune system. Could the electromagnetic force field of clocks on the nightstand be memory robbers as well? What about telephones? How many of us "live" on the phone and expose our brains to this type of electromagnetic force field? What about computers? The U.S. government recommends that no more than 2.5 milligauss should be endured for any extended period of time; however, the average computer monitor generates between 8 and 25 milligauss, depending on its size and complexity. The computer power unit itself adds another 5 to 25 milligauss. Of course, other added electrical computer devices will add even more. What negative impacts are these force fields having on the brain's gentle electric currents?

If any of these questions ring a bell in your head, sit tight. Brain and memory research in the last twenty years has made significant progress in our favor. Science knows more about memory and how to save it than it ever did before. You no longer have to live in fear. Today, there are a number of ways to treat simple forgetfulness. That's what this book is all about.

Dr. Lynda Toth and I have combined clinical experience with the most up-to-date brain research to remove the ignorance and dread many people suffer when they realize that they can't remember simple life events. We want to put your mind at ease. There are significant ways to protect and improve your memory. Important findings show that normal memory loss often can be restored and, in many cases, prevented altogether.

Part One of this book will help you understand in simple terms just how the brain gives us memory. Everyday memory loss can strike anyone if the brain function is compromised. Both conventional and unsuspected causes of memory loss are discussed in Part One. You'll see how toxic chemical exposure, poor diet and subtle nutritional deficiencies, yeast overgrowth, viral assault, heavy metal buildup, allergies, dental amalgam leakage, and a number of other causes may be robbing you of your precious memory.

Next, you'll learn how to spot problems in memory function through a series of short surveys designed to pinpoint the degree of your forgetfulness. You will come away with a clearer idea of what might be causing a loss of memory in you or in someone around you.

For instance, a pregnant woman who is experiencing bouts of memory loss during her pregnancy will discover that she can expect her memory to return to normal after the baby's delivery. This is because her hormone levels, which fluctuated during pregnancy, eventually become balanced. The person embroiled in office stress can begin having memory problems due to sensory overload. The college student pulling several "all nighters" in a row might begin losing moments of significant memory for a few days. Or the sports athlete who sweats out too many important vitamins and minerals without adequate nutrient replacement, may, over time, experience foggy, confused thinking that is characterized by an inability to recall key moments or facts.

In Part Two, you'll learn strategies to prevent and, in many cases, restore memory loss before it goes too far in your life. Even if you are not experiencing memory problems, such preventive strategies are valuable. This innovative section will give you the tools to start protecting the delicate blood-brain barrier that is so important for normal brain function and memory preservation.

Thus, a little knowledge of how your brain functions and how your memory works is beneficial. However, the real change factor will be a willingness on your part to take charge of your life and create an environment that nurtures and protects your memory. It's important to remember that Alzheimer's disease represents only one cause of memory loss—and one that constitutes only a very small percentage of cases. Other causes, which are discussed in this book, are more likely to be the reasons for memory lapses. Unfortunately, these more common causes are often unknown or simply neglected.

Memory loss is a problem you can deal with in a rational manner. But you must be willing to look at your lifestyle, become your own medical detective, and accept coaching from a doctor who is experienced in treating the causes of memory loss.

Part One

Understanding Memory

*B*rain function is like an ever-turning wheel. It never stops until one dies. Whether awake or asleep, the brain's job is to direct the chemical and electrical processing of information signals about the world. Such diverse decisions as how fast the heart needs to beat, when to send in the immune police to "fix" a wound, or how to ask for a slice of strawberry pie are all in a day's work for this major organ of the central nervous system.

So complex is the brain's coordination activity, that thousands of brain-directed activities are always going on at the same moment. In a generalized manner, you could say most of the brain is taken up with learning and memory activity. Consider the following:

- Half of all the body's nerve cells are located in the brain.

- The brain uses 25 percent of the body's energy to conduct mental and physical acts.

- Despite its many powers, the brain makes up only 2 percent of total body weight.

- The brain reacts in $1/30$ of a second to incoming signals, such as a loud noise or a visual cue.

- Current estimates tally the total number of nerve cells for the brain at 100 billion. Each microscopic nerve cell shares information with up to 10 thousand other tiny nerve cells. As a result, the brain may contain 60 trillion bits of memory.

As you read the pages of Part One, you will discover the amazing powers of the brain and the foundation for memory. You'll learn how memory works and why it sometimes fails. The workings of the human brain are detailed in the chapter opener, while subsequent chapters discuss the physical basis for memory failure—the well understood causes as well as those that are lesser known.

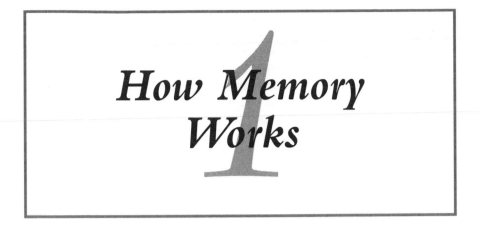

How Memory Works

*"The human brain may be the most unique organ
in the universe."*

—Dr. Arnold Scheibel
UCLA Brain Research Institute

A major concern for anyone over age forty should not be the collapse of Social Security, but whether or not he or she will enjoy the latter part of life with full memory function. The problem is that after twenty-five years of age, memory cells known as *neurons* begin to die inside your brain at the rate of up to 1 percent each year. This means you will lose about 10 percent of your total memory capability for normal thought processing between the ages of twenty-six and forty. At this rate, you are likely to lose nearly 30 percent of your total memory mass by age seventy. We are not speaking about the abnormal memory loss associated with Alzheimer's disease, a serious type of dementia. We are referring only to the everyday memory loss associated with aging.

There are a number of causes of memory loss—above and beyond those that occur as part of the natural aging process. For example, a nutrient-deficient diet can result in blood that is too weak to provide the protein building blocks needed to support memory. Also, those who have experienced oxygen depletion to the brain—the result of head trauma, strokes, or other cerebrovascular diseases—or those who have long endured the harmful effects of diabetes, thyroid dysfunction, brain infection, or stress commonly experience varying degrees of memory loss. The free radical damage resulting from alcohol, drug, or tobacco abuse also brings additional damage to one's memory, as well as the destructive force of heavy metals like mercury and nickel that come from dental amalgams and aluminum that leaches out of pots and pans. Parasitic infections, mold allergies, yeast overgrowth, and microscopic organisms, along with surgical anesthesia and prescription or recreational drugs can also have a direct impact on memory. Since each of these harmful effects of memory probably adds to the other, it is easy to understand why some people lose memory faster than others of the same age.

MEMORY LOSS IS NOT INEVITABLE

The good news is you can increase the strength of the memory neurons you still have. While brain mass does shrink in size with normal aging, it is possible to physically increase the receiving stations located on your remaining memory cells to offset normal losses. This growth potential is known as *plasticity*, and it happens each time your brain receives new sensory information. You see, learning enlarges the physical density of these branch-like ends of memory cells during a new sensory experience. This means memory connections are strengthened when you learn something you did not know before, make a new friend, or experience new surroundings. Such plasticity, or change, happens even if you are 100 years old. Once an experience becomes routine, this growth no longer occurs. The important point is that plasticity compensates for neurons lost during the normal aging process. That's why older people who want to resist the effects of time need a stimulating life environment.

That's not all. Research published in March of 1998 shattered the long-held belief that whole, complete neurons grow only in the developing fetus before birth. Important findings in animal studies show evidence of new memory cell growth in the brains of mammals similar to human beings. This neuron growth potential astounded researchers. More study is needed to discover just how new memory cell growth can be encouraged in humans on a large scale. The mere potential, however, offers considerable hope that premature memory loss, as well as Alzheimer's and other debilitating neurological diseases will be stamped out in the future.

In the meantime, there is much you can do to protect and restore your memory function before it is too late. Despite the unsettling Alzheimer's statistics, it is important to keep a positive attitude, because memory loss that comes with normal aging does not always happen. In fact, it is possible that the inability to remember as people grow older is probably unnatural and may be linked to environmental factors that might have been controlled or reversed in the patient's life.

Sound too good to be true? Meet ninety-five year old Michael of St. Louis, Missouri, who remembers seeing D.W. Griffith's famous motion picture *Birth of a Nation* in 1912. After the movie, young Michael and his family were invited to a party where they met Lillian Gish, the film's leading lady. After pasting a postage stamp of Mr. Griffith on a card, Michael asked Miss Gish for her autograph, which she gladly gave him. He still has this special souvenir and cherishes the memory of America's first Hollywood female star to this day. Don't forget, Michael is only five years away from his century birthday, yet he demonstrates normal memory. In fact, Michael is amazed when he hears of sixty- and seventy-year-olds who have memory problems. He himself has no trouble remembering new friends, new facts, or new events in his life. He finishes his sentences and does not confuse today with yesterday. Nor does Michael repeat statements every few seconds.

Why does Michael still have normal memory? A strong hint comes from the sheer variety of new sensory input he willingly accepts into his awareness each day. This active ninety-five-year-old takes a lively interest in life and has a busy social schedule with his friends, many who are under age thirty-five. Michael's admirers line up for invitations to his tea parties, which include carefully placed silverware, fresh flowers, and cloth napkins. Michael is careful to eat a balanced diet of fresh nutritious foods regularly. He gets plenty of rest and takes important nutritional supplements that feed his memory. Life is not over for Michael. He says, "My glass is half full, not half empty."

Yes, your memory can be good in your later years. Like Michael, you too can be capable of remembering the important details of your life. But you do need to mobilize a plan for memory retention or restoration now, before you get any older. Nothing happens without action. So, if you are concerned about your memory, you have made a good start in picking up this book. By the time you complete this chapter, you will have a better idea of what memory is. By the time you finish this book, you'll have specific knowledge to map out your own memory maintenance strategy.

WHAT IS MEMORY?

Memory involves the way new knowledge is saved and brought into use in everyday life. An extension of learning, your memory is made up of everything you have experienced and remembered since your conception in the womb to the present moment. Before birth, a steady, loud heartbeat told you that your mother was there. As a child, raindrops on the window meant you couldn't play outside. As a teenager, no date for the prom signaled you wouldn't be needing a new dress or tuxedo. The first day on the job after graduation, you may have felt that you weren't qualified. After retirement, you can look back and see that you had a good life after all. Memories are the sum total of life. They make you who and what you are in the world.

Your Working Memory

Since memory is always being stored, how do you cope with the sheer volume of new, moment-to-moment information throughout life? That's where *working memory* comes to your rescue. Lasting only a few seconds, your working memory quickly disappears to save storage space for more important details. The following example demonstrates how it happens.

Imagine you are about to come to an intersection when you see a car entering at the same time you are. You know the other car could hit you, so your working memory gages your speed, reminds you there's a vehicle ahead, and urges you to take action. You step on your brakes, slow down, and allow the car in the intersection to pass. When safe, you proceed down the street where another driving situation now demands attention. Up ahead, the traffic light turns yellow. You consider running it, until you see a policeman in the rearview mirror. You slow to a stop. Again, working memory has handled the moment. The dangerous situation at the previous intersection has been forgotten. Now, you are concentrating on avoiding a traffic ticket from the officer behind you. Within seconds, you will forget this experience as well, and be on to the next one. All the previous moments of working memory will be pushed into the past.

Short-Term and Long-Term Memory

If working memory needs to be retained for several minutes,

hours, or even days, *short-term memory* takes over to store this information. Facts like the plumber's phone number, how to get to your daughter's next soccer game, or what time your dental appointment is tomorrow do not matter in the overall scheme of life. Your short-term memory function knows this because the *cerebral cortex* or intelligence center, located at the top of your brain, has communicated this to the *limbic system.* The limbic system is a cluster of neurons deep inside the center of your brain that are linked with various emotions and feelings. As your emotional memory center, the limbic system coordinates incoming message information with the cortex—a layer of cells that covers the cerebrum—makes a decision about the "feelings" connected to that message, and signals a response back to the cortex.

It is not by chance that the cortex has been called your "thinking cap." It is responsible for virtually all thoughts. This shallow layer of beige nerve cells covering the cerebrum appears grooved and bumpy. Stretched out, the cortex measures about two and one-half square feet. Without the cerebral cortex, you'd be like a zombie—unable to think, feel, remember, or create a "dirty, rotten, awful" ice cream sundae and enjoy it.

This main cognitive control area has decided the plumber's phone number is not worth saving as permanent memory. Nor is your recent trip to the antique dealer (unless you made a fantastic buy). Thought centers in the frontal and temporal lobes of your cerebrum understand that some details have to be cleared away for more important memory work. Short-term memory probably evolved to save even more space for the important details of your experiences, the facts that need to be stored for the rest of your life. This is where *long-term memory* stored for days, years, even decades comes into the picture. What you learned long ago in day-to-day living is still with you in your cortex. It is made up of all the emotional and factual information your intelligence center decided to save many years ago to help you live a long life. Long-term memory also gives continuity to life and helps you develop a specific personality. The sum total of what you know is a collection of all the bits of long-term memory ever stored in your head.

Long Ago and Far Away

In the movie *Titanic,* 100-year-old Rose Calvert fails to remember that she has introduced her granddaughter to the treasure seekers only moments earlier. Her short-term memory does not allow her to recall the incident. Then, when asked if there was anything she wanted, she answered, "I'd like to see my drawing." Her long-term memory of a simple sketch drawn in her youth has helped Rose understand why she is on the exploration boat to begin with.

Once Rose sees the drawing, she begins to recall the story of her experience on the *Titanic*. Her long-term memory is crystal clear. "It's been eighty-four years, and I can still smell the fresh paint. The china had never been used . . ." Rose then proceeds to verbalize her recollection of the trip, complete with details of feelings, colors, shapes, and conflicts.

Short-term memory is very fragile in the aging brain. It is "the first to go" as brain membranes weaken with time's assault from the outside world. Long-term memory, on the other hand, tends to stay intact in most people. Only in the latter stages of Alzheimer's disease do long-term memories disappear.

Memory involves the way in which knowledge is acquired, saved, and brought from storage when needed. Such recall shows how past learning is connected to today's actions, even if such incidents happened long ago. To a great degree, long-term memory has shaped who you are and how you respond to your experiences. Long-term memories make up what you know about the world. The fact that some are negative doesn't matter. What's important is that you remember them. The contrast between the pleasure and the pain of these memories gives you a boundary of awareness called learning.

YOUR BRAIN

Before discussing memory any further, it is important to take a brief look at the place where memories are made and stored—the brain.

The functions of the brain are no less than remarkable. The most intricate computer cannot even come close to matching its capabilities. The brain is the body's control center. Thoughts, moods, memories, and behavior are all controlled by this powerful organ. It is where the centers for speech, hearing, touch, smell, and sight are located. The brain has three major components: the brain stem, the cerebellum, and the cerebrum, as seen in Figure 1.1.

Located at the base of the brain, the *brain stem* attaches the brain to the spinal cord. Critical body functions that are automatically regulated by the brain stem include breathing and heartbeat. If you had only this part of the brain, you would be like a reptile with no tendency toward love or other feelings.

The *cerebellum* lies just behind the brain stem at the back of the head. It maintains specialized memory for motor skills, helping the body make smooth, accurate movements. Athletes get their great physical coordination from this area.

The rest of the brain mass is known as the *cerebrum*, which is divided into two halves or hemispheres—the right and left. The cerebrum houses most of the capabilities for thinking and intelligence. The right side of the cerebrum governs aspects of creativity and nonverbal communication, while the left side is responsible for logical thinking and written and verbal expression. The hemi-

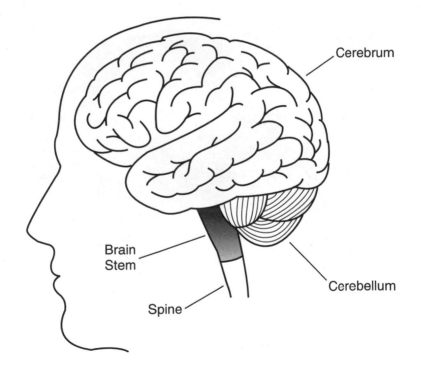

Figure 1.1. The Brain

spheres are connected by the *corpus callosum* and covered by the layer of cells known as the cortex.

As seen in Figure 1.2, the cerebrum is further divided into the temporal, frontal, parietal, and occipital lobes—each of which controls a variety of functions. Note that each lobe occurs in pairs— one in each hemisphere of the cerebrum.

The *frontal lobe* is the primary seat of memory. It allows you to engage in abstract reasoning and plan for future activity. This lobe also helps you remember to be tactful to others in social situations. It also helps you focus on an activity until it is completed. The left side of the frontal lobe is the speech center. Cells located in the back of the frontal lobe coordinate movements.

Situated beneath the frontal and parietal lobes, the *temporal lobe*

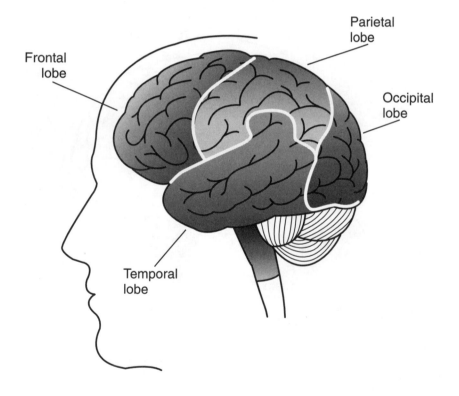

Figure 1.2. The Cerebrum

coordinates the awareness and interpretation of sounds and language. Musical skills like singing, playing an instrument, and composing are centered here. The inner surface lining of the temporal lobe integrates memories of past experiences with sights and sounds in the present. Short-term memory is held in a part of the temporal lobe called the hippocampus, which is discussed in detail beginning on page 22.

Above the cerebrum and brain stem lies the *occipital lobe*. Smaller than the other three lobes, the occipital lobe coordinates all visual activity. Nerve fibers from this lobe fan out to join many other areas of the brain in a complex "wiring system." This system offers effective protection for one's sight. Even those with severe brain damage from such causes as strokes or head trauma usually do not lose their sight.

Located at the top rear section of the cerebrum, the *parietal lobe* is a special area for the coordination of sensory information. This is where the capability for analytical reasoning and logical deduction are found. When you are working on a math problem, your parietal lobe is active. This lobe also pulls bits of information into one image in your mind. It also keeps you familiar with your surroundings. For instance, when you are leaving the mall and heading toward the parking lot, the parietal lobe calls up a mental picture of your car and connects it with memories on how to get there. Those with various kinds of dementia often have severely damaged parietal lobes, which is why these people may experience trouble finding their way home.

WHERE DOES MEMORY START?

The first time a piece of information about the outside world entered your brain through sight, sound, touch, taste, or smell, memory tissue began to lay a permanent record of the experience. Neurologists call this learning. The ability to remember began when those signals were recalled from special storage cells inside your brain.

While memory is stored throughout the brain, most people have one dominant pattern of saving their experiences. For instance, filmmaker Steven Spielberg is oriented toward visual memory and creates vivid images. For him, strong memory factors are most likely stored in his occipital lobe—the part of the brain that controls sight. Yet every time we hear the music from *Jaws*, it's obvious a lot of thinking is going on in Spielberg's temporal and frontal lobes as well.

The singing ability of Elvis Presley was strongly linked to his temporal lobe, which is responsible for musical ability. Just watch an Elvis movie and you'll see an excellent example of musical expression.

Switching gears, let's take a look at the thought activity of Albert Einstein, a renowned genius. Respected for his mathematical work on the theory of relativity, Einstein demonstrated considerable thought activity in the parietal lobe, where analytical reasoning is strong. The average Jeopardy game show contestant also has excellent parietal function. Take a look at the fine motor skills of golf wonder Tiger Woods, who, like other great athletes, exhibits special ability to store memory in his cerebellum. His physical coordination displays thought transfer that is going on in his temporal lobe, as well.

Do not get the idea these people fail to store memory in other areas of their brain. Findings at the UCLA Brain Research Institute and the University of California at Berkeley show memory gets processed in many places in the brain all at once. Information retrieval in the above examples simply shows how a particular memory area dominates because of unique talents.

Because a single memory is saved in a number of places throughout the cerebral tissue, you do not have to relearn simple tasks each morning to survive the day. Well-functioning memory also helps you "course correct" future actions and stay on target in life. By adulthood, your collection of memories will have shaped who you are. It will show where you have been in life, and provide you with a strong support structure for personality.

Explicit and Implicit Memory

The memory of Grandma's kitchen is an example of conscious or *explicit memory* because you can recall the experience whenever you want. Such memory is like having your own personalized time machine vessel that allows you to "time travel" between the present and the past. It gives you tremendous power to shape and control your environment. As far as we know, only human beings store explicit memory information. More simple forms of animal life are guided by rote instinct and live only in the moment.

The other type of recall, *implicit memory,* is more subtle because of its unconscious nature. This kind of information is stored in the basal ganglia—structures deep near the center of the brain that help regulate physical coordination. In the Tiger Woods example, implicit memory also supports conditioned reflexes and physical skills operated through the cerebellum. There is an automatic tone to implicit memory, because it carries out functions such as breathing, blood clotting, and cell repair without conscious thought.

Implicit memory also helps the brain select which physical and emotional reactions to make as it interprets sensory input. Consider how implicit memory swings into action when you accidentally cut your finger, for instance. Messenger cells in the wound area notify your brain's implicit memory with lightning speed. "There's a problem down here," is the clarion call. In a split second, the immune police rush to the area to sanitize the wound. Next, cellular repair functions take over. At the same time, fibrinogen in the blood starts clotting, and once the bleeding is brought under control, healing can begin.

All of this emergency work is conducted without conscious thought and demonstrates how implicit memory protects us despite its unconscious nature. As powerful as explicit memory, implicit memory holds everything the brain and body need to know about keeping you alive through functions such as organ operation, cell function, motor skills, habits, and reflex learning.

The Autonomic Nervous System

Implicit memory response in the *autonomic* branch of the peripheral nervous system involves many involuntary functions, including bodily repair functions, heartbeat, breathing, and digestion. This regulatory portion of the nervous system controls body organs without your conscious knowledge. A mystery for many years, today the autonomic nervous system stands center stage in studies that deal with the connection between stress and illness. This system reacts with the adrenal glands, keeping a silent memory record that helps fuel your muscles if it becomes necessary for you to stay and "fight" or run and "flee" from a dangerous situation.

Remember your first big job interview? You know, the really important one that gave you a chance to make a tremendous change in your life? You can probably still remember how dry your mouth was, how clammy your hands felt, and how hard your

heart was pounding as you neared the room in which the interview was to be held. This stress you were feeling was perceived in
the *sympathetic branch* of the autonomic nervous system.

The *parasympathetic branch* of the autonomic nervous system
regulates the opposite kind of function—the quiet ongoing processes of temperature regulation, resting, and digestion. Though
you were frightened that day of the big interview, your heart did
not stop beating nor were you unable to breathe. In fact, once the
interview was over, you probably felt great. Though subtle, various parts of the human nervous system help us get through difficult moments.

Working Hand in Hand

Although explicit memory and implicit memory are very different,
they often work hand in hand to help you survive. For instance,
explicit memory allows you to appreciate the pistachio ice cream
you're eating, while your implicit memory automatically tells your
stomach to break it down. Implicit memory also signals the pancreas to convert sugar to energy, and it promotes fat storage of any
calories that you don't burn off.

Now, let's imagine a more life-threatening situation. You are on
safari in Africa when your sensory awareness screams, "Rhino!
Rhino attacking!" Implicit memory directs your adrenal glands to
instantly pump stress hormones, cortisol and adrenaline, into your
muscles to give you that extra bit of leg power to run away.
Explicit memory will see to it that you select a big tree in which
you climb to safety.

UNRAVELING THE SECRET TO MEMORY

Only recently are scientists and researchers beginning to understand memory function. In the past, people thought emotions and
feelings were centered in the heart. While archeologists believe a
simple type of brain surgery was performed more than 4,000 years
ago in Egypt, it took the exploratory work of French physician
Paul Broca to discover that the ability to talk is located in the
brain's left frontal lobe.

Scientists, however, did not discover how memory is processed
and stored until the late 1940s. That's when Dr. Wilder Penfield
triggered memory recall in epileptic patients by stimulating specif-

ic neurons in the temporal lobe. Dr. Penfield also noticed that these patients experienced the sounds of music that they had not heard in years. Researchers were excited because they began to see a pattern of memory storage. There was, however, much they still did not understand about message processing.

Even in the 1950s and 1960s, medical science lacked the ways and means to pin down important memory function. Brain imaging techniques were little help. X-rays, for instance, were able to produce only a flat, black and white, overall image of the inside of the brain. And surgery could not reveal new information about memory because the person was unconscious during the procedure. Even when special tissue scanning devices like computerized axial tomography (CAT) and magnetic resonance imaging (MRI) scans were developed to explore brain anatomy, neurologists still had only limited knowledge of memory processes.

It took the development of the positron emission transmission (PET) scan in the 1980s to really open the door to memory function. Made for unlocking the secrets of memory processing, this "turn of the century" piece of equipment allows researchers to track and record which memory centers get stimulated in live, working brain tissue during memory processing. Some call PET scans "real time" images.

During a PET scan, a radioactive substance is injected into the bloodstream. This substance is followed as works it way into brain structures to measure brain activity. A PET scan, for instance, may show which part of the brain is most active when a person is analyzing a math problem. The computerized color imaging of a PET scan is known as *brain mapping*. Active areas of the brain—areas in which thinking and/or emotional or memory activity is taking place—show up red. Inactive areas register blue.

While there are varying theories on how we remember things, these new fact-finding tools have chipped away at the mystery of the memory process. In fact, during the last ten years, researchers have probably accumulated more knowledge about memory than they did during the previous 5,000 years. It is no wonder the 1990s are known as the "decade of the brain."

WHERE IS MEMORY STORED?

The world is so big. Your brain is so small. There is so much information to be processed and saved that the central nervous system has organized your memory in clever and intricate ways. Not long ago, neurologists thought memory was stored in just one area of the brain. But now, with the help of PET scans, they have learned memory is stored throughout many regions of the cerebrum. Just as your television receives programming from a centralized system of cable, network, and local television, your brain has a variety of memory areas that process and send out stored information to the cortex.

A tiny fragment of a specific memory is held in an individual neuron. But the entire memory is kept in the network of *memory traces*—long nerve chains that connect with various parts of the brain. Scientists still do not know exactly how a neuron retains memory. With today's knowledge, however, neurologists believe a tiny part of memory gets "laid down" or "created" when sensory input enters your awareness. This signal is carried along memory nerve cells by chemical and electrical forces. Memory input chemically changes the ribonucleic acid (RNA) of the neuron targeted for storing the memory—this means the nerve cell now holds important codes for genetic transmission. This process is believed to create genetic memory, allowing humans to pass on certain personality traits to their children. (Ever hear the saying, "The apple doesn't fall far from the tree."?)

The Limbic System—Pathway to Long-Term Memory

In order for memory to be stored, it needs a connecting mechanism between short- and long-term memory. It finds this link by way of the limbic system.

An important center for learning and memory coordination, the limbic system is located deep in the brain beneath the cerebrum. It is made up of the hippocampus, the amygdala, the hypothalamus, the thalamus, and the pituitary. Each of these specialized neuron clusters has a distinct function that supports all cognition and memory. When a sensory signal registers in your mind, its message content is analyzed by these various parts.

The first base of memory is the *hippocampus*. Short-term memory is stored here until a decision is made whether or not to ship it to long-term storage in the cortex (outer lining) of the cerebrum. Shaped like a sea horse, the hippocampus focuses on conscious memory of "unemotional" data—events, places, and facts. If there is any emotion attached to a memory signal, the impulse is sent to the amygdala.

Problems with short-term memory signify the hippocampus is damaged in some way. The continued presence of the stress hormones cortisol and adrenaline, for instance, weaken the hippocampus no matter what the person's age. College students have been known to develop temporary short-term memory problems when undergoing stress due to prolonged exams or concern over grades. Damage to the hippocampus can also be the result of the herpes virus, which has been known to attack this area. Low levels of key neurotransmitters are also believed to weaken neurons in the hippocampus.

Any damage to the hippocampus will result in short-term memory loss. This is why elderly people—during the normal aging process—may tend to lose short-term memory, while retaining details from their distant past. Long-term memory, which is stored in the cortex, tends to resist loss. Yet, any cellular attack on hippocampal neurons—from aging or the other causes just mentioned—will result in short-term memory lapses.

The second base for memory is the *amygdala*. Any information with emotional content is sent to the amygdala by the hippocampus for analysis. The amygdala is an almond-shaped collection of master neurons located deep in the brain's temporal lobe. Though poorly understood in the past, the amygdala is now attracting worldwide interest from neurologists. By acting as an assistant to the hippocampus in the storage of information, the amygdala is the main switching station for your innermost feelings. Call it emotion central.

Remember the first time you had a "crush" on someone in elementary school? Or that first valentine you received from someone special? Such emotional memories have been coordinated by your amygdala, then sent to the cortex for long-term storage. That's why you can remember emotional feelings from the past. The evolution of this part of the limbic system helped early human beings protect their young. Scientists believe the evolutionary development of the amygdala also led to social interaction and increased cooperation in human societies.

Scent memory is also coordinated and saved by the amygdala. Ever notice how a particular smell can trigger a vivid memory? Perhaps the aroma of warm bread triggers the memory of Grandma's kitchen, while the smell of roasted garlic reminds you of your first dinner in a fancy restaurant. Memories are often far more powerful when a particular scent stimulates recall because they are interlinked through the amygdala. If your amygdala were removed, you would not experience feelings toward anything.

The third base in memory processing is the *hypothalamus*. This important part of the limbic system controls sexual function, thirst, sleep cycles, the autonomic system, emotions, body temperature, immunity, weight control, and all sorts of biological "clocks" in the body. The hypothalamus is easily damaged by biochemical upsets in the brain—upsets, for instance, caused by flavor enhancers in processed foods. Acting as a regulator of hormone ratios, the hypothalamus is fragile because, unlike other parts of the limbic system, it lacks the protective membrane known as the blood-brain barrier (page 29). Without this membrane, toxins in the blood more easily infiltrate the area, contributing to inflammatory damage of the hypothalamus, possibly setting the stage for serious memory diseases later in life.

Although involved in the memory process, the hypothalamus does not come into play until the hippocampus, amygdala, and cortex of the cerebrum have assigned a ranked importance to the situation or memory at hand. Once the hypothalamus gets this message, it passes the signal over to the pituitary. During times of alarm, the hypothalamus screams for help from your adrenal glands. Almost instantly, the stress hormones cortisol and adrenaline surge to the neurons to give them extra power for the emergency.

As long as memory neurons are not constantly subjected to cortisol, there is no damage to memory. However, too much cortisol over a long period of time can damage the neurons. This is because excess cortisol floods the neuron bodies and memory pathways with too much calcium. Though necessary for memory, calcium is supposed to stay only a short while before being reabsorbed out of the memory pathway. Constant bombardment of cortisol causes eventual neuron death.

The *thalamus* is the limbic system's public address system. It sends all incoming sensory information to various places in the brain, linking different parts of the limbic system to each other. This is why memory is not stored in just one spot. The one sensory message the thalamus does not process is smell. That job, as mentioned previously, is performed by the amygdala.

And last, but not least, is the tiny *pituitary*. This gland is the prime controller for hormone activity in the endocrine system. As an umpire calls the shots in baseball, the pituitary gland tells other endocrine glands which hormones to secrete and when. High levels of pituitary secretions in the blood signify that the thyroid gland is not secreting enough of its hormone. This is important, because certain thyroid conditions can contribute to poor memory if left untreated.

Tracing a Message Impulse

To better understand how memory connects to various parts of the brain, let's imagine you see the classic 1950s movie *Some Like It Hot*. You especially like one of the scenes in which Marilyn Monroe dances. You like her steps and practice them until you know them by heart. Meeting a friend, you show him the dance, chattering on about how great you think Marilyn was in the movie.

A PET scan of your brain at this moment would show activity in the cortex (the memory center that records facts, people, and places). It is the cortex that knows you are thinking about a movie, not the real Marilyn. It also remembers the theater in which you saw the movie, the day you saw it, and whether or not you liked the popcorn.

Since you admire Marilyn and have strong admiration for her, your amygdala (the center for emotional memory) would also show activity. The hippocampus has decided this intense feeling is worth keeping, so it ships the memory of Marilyn and her dance to the cortex for long-term storage. As you perform the dance steps you learned from the movie, memory in your cerebellum would be active, because this is where your motor memory ability is located. But the overall skill you learned in duplicating her dance steps is being stored in the memory neurons of the basal ganglia of your cerebral cortex. Each of these memory areas will be activated every time you think about Marilyn Monroe.

THE PHYSICAL WORKINGS OF MEMORY

Like Butch Cassidy, a *neuron* is the leader and "decision maker" in the path of memory. *Glia cells*, on the other hand, are reminiscent of the Sundance Kid because they ride shotgun to neurons by supporting their life and activity. Three parts of the neuron are crucial in the flow of memory as it moves from one end of the cell body to the other. These parts are the dendrite, the cell body, and the axon, shown in Figure 1.3.

The message-receiving part of a neuron is the *dendrite*. A memory neuron has many of these antenna-like branches on the cell body. Each dendrite is studded with thousands of minute spines to help perceive and process memory. It is through these tiny dendrite branches and spines that billions of thought and memory processes work together every moment you are alive and using your brain.

No matter how young or old you are, dendrites are capable of rapid growth and extension. The more dendrites you have the better your memory. Every time you learn something new in life or experience a different sensation, additional dendrite receiving stations sprout and grow to further accommodate new knowledge. The growth of dendrites through lifelong learning can prolong your memory capacity no matter what age you are. This may mean learning to play the piano at age seventy, traveling to Alaska at eighty, or studying opera at ninety. This is why it is so important to constantly seek out new and unique experiences to stimulate and enrich the growth of existing neurons. In short, never roll over and say to yourself, "I'm too old." Such thinking is bad for memory, and it has nothing to do with the truth about memory formation.

The second important part of a neuron is the *cell body*. Herein lies the command center that regulates memory flow. Besides holding the genetic code for the cell, this main neuron trunk produces energy in a cell furnace called the *mitochondria*. In order to power

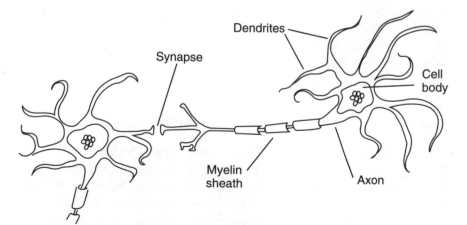

Figure 1.3. Parts of a Neuron

all thought and memory activity, these energy furnaces use 20 percent of the total oxygen taken into the body every second of your life. One-fourth of all of your blood sugar is also used to produce energy in the mitochondria. This is a great consumption of energy for an organ that makes up only 2 percent of the entire body weight. It is an amazing ratio that shows the importance of energy in your memory function. Even when you are under anesthesia, the cell body of a neuron still consumes huge quantities of energy. Some of this power generates the electricity, which moves memory through the cell body. The rest is used for other memory activity. The bottom line is that your brain must meet its moment-by-moment energy needs. If it cannot, neurons grow weak and begin to die. When this happens, you will begin to notice that you cannot remember things as well as you once did.

The final component of a neuron is the *axon*—the sending station of memory. Each axon is surrounded by a *myelin sheath*, a kind of insulator that acts very much like the insulation surrounding an electrical wire. Fifty years of research has finally revealed the mystery of how memory moves through the various parts of the brain. In a process known as the *axon potential*, an amazing blend of electrical and chemical energy moves memory from one neuron to millions of others.

Normally, messages are transmitted in one direction—from the axon of one neuron to the dendrite of the next. But bioelectricity cannot carry the signal across the *synapse*—the microscopic gap found between neurons. In order to bridge this space, neurons make use of special biochemical "go-betweens" that are produced in the neuron body. These chemical substances are known as *neurotransmitters*, and they piggyback memory information to the next neuron by surging into the synaptic gap. When the electrical charge pushes the message through the neuron and it reaches the axon, neurotransmitters are released into the synaptic space. Now, the memory signal has a chemical bridge by which it can travel to the nearby dendrite receiving stations. For detailed information on specific neurotransmitters, see the discussion beginning on page 41.

You might be wondering why the synapse exists. The answer lies in versatility. Without the gap, memory would not be able to make the rapid changes and adjustments in response to the various information signals. Synapses help you and your memory survive in a hostile world.

The Glia Cell—The Sundance Kid of Memory

What about the neuron's sidekick, the *glia cell*? Serving as a kind of glue for neurons, glia cells help hold the memory path together by regulating the concentration of mineral ions, such as potassium, sodium, and calcium that trigger an electrical charge. Glia cells outnumber neurons ten to one and serve as their caretakers, supporting and nourishing them. Glia cells generally lack synapses and cannot process or store a memory impulse, as do neurons. But they reproduce themselves much more easily than neurons. Together, memory neurons and glia cells carry you on a big memory adventure throughout life. That's why we call them the Butch Cassidy and Sundance Kid of memory.

HOW IS A MEMORY CREATED?

Specialized bundles of nerve cells that work in conjunction with each other, neurons are designed to carry sensory messages throughout the brain and spinal cord. Think for a moment about the first time you learned the name of a new friend. Maybe you repeated the name over and over to make sure you wouldn't forget it. The first time you heard the name, the sensory information passed through one of your neurons slowly. Each time you repeated the name, the memory imprint got stronger as it moved through the neuron. Finally, after repeated travels, the memory signal was able to shoot very quickly across synapses and through neuronal tissue when called up from memory.

What happens in the synaptic space between neurons is very important for memory. As discussed earlier, in order to bridge this tiny gap, neurotransmitters "piggy back" memory messages to the dendrites on the next neuron, and the one after that, and so on.

The more dendrite branches you have, the better your memory. This is because more information will be moving at the same time. But you also need sufficient amounts of these chemical message carriers to keep memory working across synapses between memory cells. When neurotransmitters drop in concentration, memory weakens and you start saying, "I don't remember."

Health of a Neuron

Since the presence of neurotransmitters in the synapse also triggers another spurt of electricity in the stem of the neuron, memory will continue to move toward another dendrite where more neurotransmitters carry it across the next synapse. Once the job of these chemical message carriers is done, they are reabsorbed out of the synaptic space.

This process continues until the memory information gets to its destination. Leftover neurotransmitter substance must be cleared up by its own absorption factor to protect receptors in the synapse. As always, maintaining a proper balance among all forces in memory tissue is a delicate issue. Too few or too many neurotransmitters can hamper the memory environment. For instance, the neurotransmitter glutamate is necessary to clear ammonia—the harmful metabolic waste product—out of memory cells. Yet, if glutamate levels get too high from dietary sources, neurons get inflamed and eventually die.

To offset this effect, each neurotransmitter has a "cleanup" enzyme to pull it out of the synapse to prevent burnout. For instance, the enzyme acetylcholinesterase pulls excess acetylcholine out of the synapse until the next memory comes along. If neurotransmitter regulation is disrupted, the result is neuronal death. In fact, this is how some pesticides and warfare chemicals work. By destroying the proper balance of acetylcholine, the nervous system of a host organism is knocked out of commission. This neurotransmitter disruption, in either an insect or a soldier on a battlefield, causes nerve paralysis of the respiratory system. The final result is a total shutdown of all bodily functions and death.

Memory function is very complex. Imagine this process duplicated trillions of times every second in every memory cell in your head. It is mind-boggling to consider how many chemical and electrical processes go on in your brain during the period of one day. Crucial nutrient building blocks must be present for this flow of information through neurons. Such organic materials are obtained through powerful enzymes in food, mostly raw food. In most cases, the more raw food you eat, the more memory-building enzymes you will have for good memory.

Blood-Brain Barrier—The Ultimate Memory Armor

In the ancient fable *Ali Baba and the Forty Thieves,* a fantastic treasure was stored in a cave and protected behind a magic door. Only certain words would permit entry. Like Ali Baba's magic door, the blood-brain barrier guards the inner structure of most neurons. Made up of a dual layer of cells that fit tightly on the outside of the neuron bodies, the blood-brain barrier allows only certain electrons and molecules to pass through it to the cerebral stores of memory neurons. This selective membrane keeps out harmful toxins and disease-causing organisms that prevent learning and memory retention.

But when foreign substances like heavy metals, such as those commonly found in smog or polluted water, weaken and penetrate the blood-brain barrier, the flow of memory suffers. The membrane layer of this protective barrier loses its tight "fit," and is unable to effectively protect the memory-processing neurons. This creates havoc in brain tissue. Neurotransmitter levels in the memory cells are disturbed, genetic blueprints destroyed, and inflammation starts burning up neurons. Free radical oxidation increases as a vicious death cycle picks up speed in memory tissue.

There are four areas of the brain that do not develop a blood-brain barrier. These unprotected areas of memory include the hypothalamus, the circumventricular organs, the pineal body, and the locus ceruleus—a small cluster of nerves in the brain stem.

Without a reliable blood-brain barrier, neurons are at the mercy of destructive forces. First, there is dwindling protection for working- and short-term memory. And as lesions increase, even long-term memory will be affected. Thus, it is crucial to protect the blood-brain barrier. It is equally important to minimize the toxic forces in the brain at large and save memory neurons in areas where no blood-brain barrier exists. Supporting the blood-brain barrier can be done in a number of ways, including reducing free radical damage, keeping brain nutrient levels high, and avoiding neurotoxic substances in foods and beverages (all of which will be discussed at length in Chapters 3 and 4).

A Dramatic New Finding

Earlier in this chapter, we mentioned the demise of a once-held belief that when a neuron dies it is gone forever. A recent joint study between researchers at Princeton University in New Jersey and Rockefeller University in New York City, involved the hippocampus tissue of monkeys. The results of the study indicate that these higher primates are able to grow not just new dendrites, but whole new neurons. This news is very exciting because it means the beginning of the end for illnesses like Alzheimer's and Parkinson's disease. If neurologists can discover how to trigger massive neuron growth in adults, permanent damage to memory may become a thing of the past. Doctors will be able to encourage massive neuronal growth in patients with degenerative memory disease and prevent the brain damage found in age-related dementia. Although the neuron growth noted was found only in the hippocampus, researchers in the study are hopeful that, eventually, neurons can be grown elsewhere in memory tissue.

Presently, no one knows how to increase neurons to match their death rate in human beings. But until science finds this answer, you can help yourself by preserving and increasing the branch-like dendrites on the neurons left in your memory mass. You can also take steps to protect your memory from free radical damage and energy-related problems in neuron tissue.

We believe this is why Michael, that debonair ninety-five-year-old we discussed earlier in the chapter, continues to function as well as a younger man in matters of cognition and memory. Michael admits he avoids stress in his daily routine, eats healthy foods, avoids excessive alcohol consumption, makes an effort to meet younger people, and works at staying relaxed and calm. These are subtle but important clues to Michael's brain longevity and healthy memory function.

Though he has probably lost some memory mass, Michael's desire to experience new activities in life continues to encourage new message connections between his neurons. With the recent findings that memory cells can grow long after development in the womb, Michael may even be growing new neurons! Through all of his life-enriching projects, positive attitudes, and low-stress life, Michael contributes to the longevity of the memory cells he has left. His reward is good memory.

IN SUMMARY

Because a memory can't be seen, held, tasted, smelled, or weighed, we tend to overlook its importance. Yet, memory is to awareness what wheels are to cars. Good memory takes us on a wonderful journey through life. Each second of life, memory provides the brain with an ability to perceive, store, and bring back into human awareness the information necessary for survival and enjoyment in life. This ability to reproduce learning through recall is more than mere remembrance. It shapes emotion, colors judgment, and leads to full expression of life. Whatever makes a moment immortal comes by way of an ability to remember the past in a present moment. Without memory, we would have no ability to learn from our mistakes. Human memory glues all experience into what we know as "a life."

Now that you know the foundation of how memory works, in the next chapter you'll learn why memory fails.

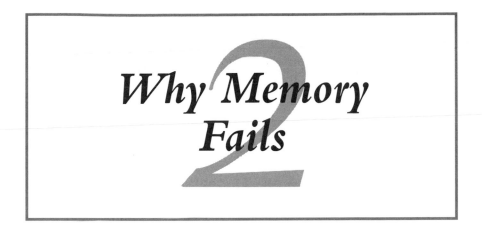

Why Memory Fails

*"One must have a good memory to be able to
keep the promises one makes."*

—F.W. Nietzche

You cross the living room and head for the kitchen. Only when you get there, you can't remember why you are there. Even worse, you can't remember things that happened yesterday without familiar reminders. And your house is full of unfinished projects because you find it difficult to concentrate long enough to complete them. Calling this your "brain fog," you ask yourself, "Why can't I remember things anymore?"

The first time a memory neuron dies in your brain, you won't be aware of it. However, when millions of neurons are damaged, you'll begin to notice memory changes. At first, you may blame it on lack of sleep, stress, or too much work. But when memory loss begins to show up with increasing frequency, you won't be able to ignore it. At this stage, many people become filled with anxiety, fearing the onset of Parkinson's or Alzheimer's disease. However, it is important to understand that memory loss can be reversed more often than not, particularly in the early stages.

The media has also played a part in adding to the fear of Parkinson's and Alzheimer's disease with its predictions of dramatic increases in the number of these cases among those born after World War II. As a result, people panic at the first sign of memory loss and assume nothing can be done to help them.

Nothing is further from the truth. Once you understand what destroys memory function, you can take action to prevent and treat its early loss. A change in lifestyle, diet, and nutrient supplementation can lessen the chance of developing serious memory problems.

A failure to process, store, and retrieve memory may be related to one or more of the following biological malfunctions in the neurons of the brain:

- Oxygen deprivation

- Low blood sugar

- Free radical damage

- Neurotransmitter depletion

- High stress levels

- Blood-brain barrier damage

Because a progressive failure to remember creates anxiety, it's important that you understand each of these factors. The choice is really up to you. How much change are you willing to undergo to reduce the risk of permanent memory loss?

If you already have significant problems associated with memory loss, such as depression, inability to concentrate, sleep disturbance, or unexplained mood swings—all possible signs of premature brain aging—the memory restoration strategies in upcoming chapters can bring positive results for you. One thing is sure. The sooner you learn what causes most memory loss, the more likely you will be motivated to protect or restore it. You can win rather than lose in the fight to save this most basic of life processes.

OXYGEN DEPRIVATION

Cells that process memory need energy just like an automobile engine. Oxygen is the ignition switch in the tiny cell furnace known as the *mitochondria*. Here, oxygen changes glucose or blood sugar into a useable cell fuel called adenosine triphosphate (ATP). This energy conversion process is called *metabolism*. Oxygen is the only substance able to change blood sugar into brain fuel. Unlike other body cells, memory neurons do not store energy. They only produce it. For this reason, the neuron is especially vulnerable to any fuel shortage because its cell body has no reserves of ATP. Thus, on a moment-to-moment basis, oxygen and sugar must always be present in brain tissue to make ATP for simple thought and memory processing.

The need for cellular fuel is so great that the brain uses 20 percent of the body's total oxygen intake to supply energy to memory neurons. Because of this need, blood circulation to the brain must never be blocked in any way. Thousands of thought and memory neurons in the cerebrum, cerebellum, and brain stem depend on ATP to power memory during every second of life. Without this cellular fuel, neurons struggle to process and interpret information.

The need to power memory with oxygen does not stop in the brain. Blood must circulate back to the lungs to get more fresh oxygen. When arterial flow is blocked by a blood clot or narrowed arterial walls, memory cells are again denied all the elements for needed energy. Such a power shortage damages the branches and roots of a neuron, and eventually the entire memory cell shrivels up and dies. If too many neurons die, memory pathways are severed.

The brain needs plenty of oxygen and glucose for optimal functioning. It is through healthy circulation that this energy cycle for memory is achieved.

LOW BLOOD SUGAR

Since normal levels of ATP energy also require blood glucose, energy levels suffer when too little sugar reaches the brain. Energy conversion for memory first starts with the digestion of carbohydrates and starches by various enzymes. These starches are then dissolved into smaller units and changed into a special sugar known as glucose, which is then absorbed into the blood. The glucose then circulates to the brain where it passes through the protective shield of the blood-brain barrier to reach neurons. Once inside the neurons, glucose changes into the energy form of ATP. As long as there is enough glucose to convert to ATP, each memory neuron has the power it needs to carry out thought and memory processing. When levels drop, however, neurons are especially vulnerable, as seen in the following example.

Fran, a popular thirty-eight-year-old high school teacher, began to experience fatigue accompanied by headaches in the late afternoon. She passed it off to the stress of teaching teenagers. By the time she reached forty, Fran noticed she was often weak and shaky just before noon. Her memory seemed to be getting worse by the month and she was experiencing feelings of sadness much of the time.

Though a standard blood test showed no evidence of a problem, Fran's doctor suspected that her symptoms were related to low blood sugar, or hypoglycemia. Commonly, people who suffer from this illness eat too many processed starches like pasta, baked goods, and snack chips. The body is forced to respond to such excessive amounts of sugar by calling up insulin from the pancreas to lower sugar levels in the blood. Because the same blood that goes through the body also circulates inside the head, memory tissue gets drained of sugar just like the rest of the body. But the brain is almost as vulnerable to decreases in sugar levels as it is to the absence of oxygen. Pulling sugar away from nerve cells inside the head is like denying a regular bottle feeding to a baby.

Fran, whose students always brought her donuts, candies, and homemade coffee cakes, was a prime candidate for low blood sugar. She regularly ate these and other highly refined carbohydrates around lunch time. While the sweets once gave her a burst of energy, just the opposite began happening. Fran noticed that she began to feel very weak and irritable after eating a candy bar. When she tried to raise her energy level with cookies, soda, or other sweets, her insulin response did just the opposite. Low sugar levels left her feeling fatigued, moody, and headachy. Too much insulin resulted in a shortage of sugar fuel for ATP energy, placing a strain on her cerebral control center. This made it difficult to keep her basic body functions going. Fran's cognitive and memory functions were left struggling for the energy to perform normal thought and mental activity on a constant basis.

Low blood sugar also put an added strain on Fran's adrenal glands by calling for more adrenaline and cortisol, which was needed to stop the insulin from letting sugar levels get to low. This pulled glucagon from her pancreas and growth hormones from her pituitary to replace low fuel levels with stored sugar in the liver. Just like falling dominos, added strain was now placed on Fran's liver.

Many complicated health processes begin to falter when the energy derived from sugar drops in the body cells. When sugar is cut off from a neuron, it has a hard time burning fat for needed energy. If low blood sugar is chronic year after year, the long-range energy loss weakens overall cognitive and memory function. In severe cases, chronic low blood sugar damages memory tissue much like oxygen deprivation does. Alzheimer's patients tend to have low blood sugar levels. Since memory cells cannot store energy, their fuel requirements operate on a narrow margin in the hippocampus—the major center for short-term memory. Denying this vulnerable area the fuel it needs to work contributes to short-term memory loss.

There is another, very frightening effect of low energy levels in the brain. Studies have shown that when neurons are depleted of fuel, they are more susceptible to damage caused by food additives like the flavor enhancers glutamic acid and L-cysteine, or aspartic acid, a sugar substitute. These substances, called *excitotoxins* by neurologists, overstimulate memory neurons. Chemical balance is all important in the health of a memory cell. In the normal, well-functioning memory cell, calcium must be able to flow in and out of the neuron body when necessary. If too much calcium floods a memory cell, special pumps push the excess out of the neuron. This extra calcium is stored in the *endoplasmic reticulum,* a parking lot for calcium that lies outside the memory pathways. Excessive amounts of excitotoxins allow the calcium channels to remain open too long. As a result, calcium remains in the neuron and the cell body cannot rest. This stimulated state results in increased inflammation. Thus, constantly eating foods with excitotoxins is like lighting a bonfire in memory cells.

Maintaining energy levels in memory neurons is one strategy to fight the damaging effects of these food additives. Be sure to read food labels, especially on items such as bottled condiments, canned goods, and bags of chips and other snacks. Beware of ingredients described on labels as "natural flavoring," "natural seasoning," "herbs," "spices," "malted barley flour," and "hydrolyzed vegetable protein." (See inset on page 67 for detailed listing of these terms.)

Do not ignore the warning signs of low blood sugar—weakness, fatigue, inability to concentrate, and vague feelings of imbalance or irritation. Meeting the basic energy requirements of memory function is crucial if you want to protect or restore memory. Like an internal combustion engine, memory neurons need the ATP fuel made from blood sugar to power sensation, process thoughts, move short-term input in long-term storage, and retrieve information. Without this energy, thought processing goes no-where. After all, the ability to think and remember is a physical process. How well your memory functions in your life depends directly on sugar and its combustion with oxygen.

FREE RADICAL DAMAGE

Larry dislikes what he sees in the mirror. Though he's only sixty-one, he looks seventy-five and feels like one hundred and one. Larry's face is etched with deep wrinkles. With little energy these days, he is moving slower all the time. But what bothers Larry most is the speed with which his mind seems to be slipping. When he got lost in public last week, he panicked and sat down on a park bench and cried until a police officer came to his rescue.

Besides living alongside a freeway, Larry is a heavy cigarette smoker. He scoffs at the idea of drinking filtered water despite warnings from the local news media about heavy metal contami-nation in the city's water supply. He doesn't like to cook, so his usual evening meal is a TV dinner, which he heats up in the micro-wave.

What Larry does not know is that rapid oxygenation—a kind of internal "rusting"—is stripping away his memory. One cause is his lack of good nutrition; the other is his exposure to environmen-tal pollutants. His cigarette smoking, his daily exposure to the heavy metals found in the air from the freeway and his tap water, and the mercury fillings in his teeth are known causes of *free radi-cals*. These lone, unstable particles are chemically reactive electrons that join readily with other compounds. Free radicals attack cells and cause damage in the body.

There are far too many sources of potential free radical damage from heavy metals and pollutants in Larry's life. Add to this a nutritionally poor diet, and Larry's middle-age body is defenseless against the burning effects of free radicals. Since the nerve cells in Larry's brain are also affected by free radicals, it is no wonder his memory is failing.

What Exactly Are Free Radicals?

Every healthy cell in your body is held together by the stable bond-ing of electrons in a marriage of molecules. But no one wants to be alone. So like Scarlett O'Hara, who stole men away from other women, "free" unpaired electrons will attack and grab a bonded electron of a healthy molecule to make its own marriage. This leaves the damaged molecule unbalanced and on the prowl for an electron it can steal from another healthy molecule. Soon a chain reaction of destruction rages in cell tissue unless certain body enzymes are present to neutralize the free radical rampage. A young body produces enough of these enzyme groups to corral and neutralize the outlaw electrons; the aging body tends to produce less.

Everyone these days wants to know how to stop these outlaws, which are found in smog, rancid fat, cigarette tars and smoke, pesticides, electromagnetic radiation, and food and water with heavy metal contaminants. Everything from cerebrovascular disease, stroke, cancer, and genetic disruption are believed to be initiated by free radicals. When these slash-and-burn chain reactions get started in your brain, neurons are destroyed in large numbers. Eventually, actual lesions or trenches can be seen in brain tissue. When free radical damage can no longer be controlled by natural body processes, they survive at the expense of memory.

Free Radicals Are Not All Bad

Strange as it may seem, free radicals are made by the immune system to fight and kill bacteria and viruses. They are also needed to produce essential hormones. Certain free radicals stimulate enzymes that make other significant chemicals for the body, such as the important blood regulators known as *prostaglandins*. Free radicals also help the body produce energy. In this function, they help cell tissue live and thrive. But free radicals must be kept in balance.

As you grow older, your body does not cope with free radicals as well as it once did. To make matters worse, there is the extra exposure to free radicals from cigarette smoke, smog, radiation, heavy metals, solvents, and pesticides in the environment. Exposure to such pollution can even speed the aging process of children.

NEUROTRANSMITTER DEPLETION

As discussed in Chapter 1, special chemical substances known as neurotransmitters exist in the brain just to carry message signals between memory neurons. Without them, memory has no vehicle in which to travel throughout the brain. Neurologists have located more than one hundred of these chemical message carriers, but only eight make a significant impact on your memory. Some neurotransmitters affect sexual arousal, others contribute to feelings of happiness or sadness. Others let you flex and contract muscles during anger or passion. Lowered amounts of neurotransmitters contribute to poor concentration, mood swings, slow thinking, and general brain fatigue.

Receptors in the synapses (spaces) between memory cells decide if a particular neurotransmitter will stimulate or inhibit thought and memory activity. But individual neurotransmitters must be in sufficient concentration to make a good memory connection for you. As these chemical carriers get used up after a while, new supplies must be made constantly from adequate levels of enzymes, trace minerals, vitamins, and amino acids, among other substances. Shortages or imbalances of neurotransmitters over a long period of time starve the neuron body and bring on its premature death. When more and more neurons disappear, brain fatigue, depression, anxiety, or forgetfulness become noticeable. By this time, the "hard wiring" of memory has been compromised beyond limits and the ability to select, store, and retrieve information will not be what it once was in your life.

Neurotransmitter Balance

An important fact about neurotransmitters is that they are in constant motion. They do not linger in memory pathways. Each neurotransmitter has a special enzyme that either pushes or pulls it from the neuron body or the synaptic gap. This mechanism is very important. Chemicals used in warfare as well as those found in pesticides paralyze the body's nervous system by preventing specific enzymes from clearing neurotransmitters from the message pathway of nerve cells. This is why warfare chemicals came to be known as "nerve gas"—they render the nervous system useless. You see, when too many neurotransmitters are left in the synaptic gap, proper signal activity is disrupted in the central nervous system. The victim's respiratory system becomes inactive, then "zap," the brain suffocates from lack of oxygen.

Life inside your central nervous system is very much a matter of balance. Too few neurotransmitters in the synaptic gap prevent proper message transmission, causing nerve damage in memory tissue. On the other hand, too many neurotransmitters in the memory pathway disrupt proper signal activity, eventually resulting in neuronal death.

Neurotransmitters That Promote Healthy Memory

Made from a variety of body enzymes, protein chains, and amino acids, neurotransmitters are responsible for the transport of millions of memory signals that move between neurons. Let's take a look at some of these important memory carriers, and see how they affect your mental function.

Acetylcholine

Considered the most important neurotransmitter for memory and thinking, acetylcholine was discovered in the early 1900s by German biochemist Otto Lowe. Important for message transmission by nerves in the brain and spinal cord, acetylcholine is released at all neuromuscular junctions and requires the amino acid choline for its biosynthesis.

Acetylcholine influences other molecules to change their forms very quickly, affecting as many as 5,000 molecules per second. Important in the storage and retrieval of memory information, acetylcholine facilitates most memory reactions. Though present throughout the brain, acetylcholine is found primarily in the hippocampus, hypothalamus, and thalamus—the important crossroads for learning, emotions, and memory. Acetylcholine levels function in a normal pattern among older people right up until they die of other causes.

Alzheimer's victims suffer from a shortage of acetylcholine. However, studies indicate that low levels of acetylcholine are only a partial cause of memory loss. Nutritional shortages and damage caused by certain food additives are other significant factors in the demise of acetylcholine.

Norepinephrine

Considered an "excitatory catecholamine," norepinephrine—also known as noradrenaline—serves memory when a strong emotion stimulates your limbic system. This neurotransmitter helps record long-term memories in the neocortex of the brain. Like acetylcholine, norepinephrine is derived from choline, but it specifically helps extra oxygen and sugar get to the brain for good memory function. Since cortisol, the chemical byproduct of stress, steals away the brain's power supply of glucose, significant levels of norepinephrine are needed to restore the brain's overall ability to store, process, and receive information.

Norepinephrine is needed especially in the hippocampus, where it helps take short-term memory and put it into long-term storage in the cortex. Too much of this neurotransmitter keeps one awake; low levels discourage a normal sex drive. The amino acids L-tyrosine and L-phenylalanine are necessary for the production of norepinephrine. Proper levels of vitamins B_3, B_6, and C, as well as the mineral copper are also necessary to produce this neurotransmitter.

Dopamine

Found primarily in the brain stem, dopamine has a calming effect on neurons and other tissue. Like most neurotransmitters and hormones, dopamine levels decrease with age. The problem is that even moderate shortages of dopamine can bring on depression, thinking dysfunction, and decreased sexual interest.

Dopamine was found to be severely lacking in the more than 500,000 patients diagnosed with Parkinson's disease in the United States. Doctors began to notice that many patients were relieved of their tremors and shaking limb muscles when dopamine levels were returned to a normal range. A synthetic form of dopamine known as levodopa (L-dopa) is given to Parkinson's patients to help balance neurotransmitter levels and control shaking muscles. Levodopa does, however, lose its effectiveness over time.

High levels of this neurotransmitter are needed to maintain normal memory, sex drive, and balanced mood levels. Dopamine also encourages the secretion of growth hormone, which is necessary for motor control.

Serotonin

Synthesized from the amino acid tryptophan, serotonin is your brain's "sunshine" neurotransmitter; it makes you feel on top of the world. Serotonin is found in many parts of the body, including blood platelets, mast cells, and digestive cells in the intestinal tract. It is also found in moderate amounts in the amygdala—the brain's emotional processing center for memory. Serotonin keeps you feeling good and helps control pain sensation.

Second only to acetylcholine as a memory neurotransmitter, serotonin prevents depression and is the precursor for melatonin, an important hormone that regulates sleep patterns. As melatonin prevents cellular changes that lead to cancer, you can see how important adequate levels of serotonin are in maintaining the delicate interplay between the nervous and immune systems.

Gamma-Aminobutyric Acid (GABA)

An inhibitory neurotransmitter needed to calm neuron receptors after memory "firing," gamma-aminobutyric acid, or GABA, exists in high concentrations throughout the central nervous system. It brings on sleep and a sense of calmness. In the brain's amygdala, GABA is found in higher concentrations than any other neurotransmitter. People with low GABA levels tend to get tense and find it hard to cope with all of the sensory stimulation coming from our technological world.

Antidepressants, such as Valium, are sometimes prescribed to help regulate the activity of GABA receptors, but there are numerous side effects to these types of drugs. It is recommended that natural substances, such as valerian root and St. John's wort, are used for calming nerves. These substances, however, are not recommended for long-term use, and they should be taken only under the approval of a qualified health-care professional.

Glutamic Acid

Found in high concentrations in the thalamus, glutamic acid is a major neurotransmitter in the brain. It is involved in storing new memories and retrieving old ones. This amino acid is important in the metabolism of sugars and fats, and aids in the transportation of potassium across the blood-brain barrier. Considered a major brain fuel, glutamic acid helps produce other amino acid transmitters in the central nervous system. Its concentration in memory tissue is up to 1,000 times higher than in other parts of the body. Along with aspartic acid, glutamic acid activates many different receptors on nerve cells. A shortage of glutamic acid causes increased levels of ammonia, a harmful oxidant that destroys memory cells.

Glutamic acid reduces brain fatigue and aids in concentration. It also activates receptors on the ends of dendrites during the memory leap across the synaptic gap between neurons. This may be why younger people who have higher levels of glutamic acid, tend to be very "quick on the draw" where memory is concerned.

In the 1980s, concern for low-levels of naturally produced glutamic acid caused some health-care practitioners to recommend this amino acid be taken in a supplemental form. Today, however, this practice is met with conflicting reactions. Many in the health-care field believe supplemental glutamic acid should be taken with caution, and only under the advisement of a qualified health-care professional. (This is especially wise considering that glutamic acid in the form of "processed free" glutamic acid is popularly added to many foods as a flavor enhancer.) The reason for this precautionary measure is that high glutamic acid levels cause the overstimulation of neurons, eventually causing their death. Recent studies show a strong correlation between high levels of dietary monosodium glutamate (MSG) and neuron destruction.

It is, therefore, wise to avoid any processed foods that contain MSG or any other excitotoxins. Glutamic acid that is produced in the body is natural and necessary. The type that is added to foods and beverages through MSG and other flavor enhancers is harmful to memory receptors because it upsets the normal concentration of the brain's natural glutamic acid.

Be sure to read food labels. Commonly used as a flavor enhancer, glutamic acid is added to foods and beverages and can be found on ingredient labels under such seemingly harmless terms as "natural flavoring" or "natural seasoning." (See inset on page 67 for detailed listing of these terms.)

Nitric Oxide

Considered the "new kid on the block," nitric oxide has been recognized as an important neurotransmitter in the last several years. Made from the amino acid L-arginine, nitric oxide does a kind of "cha cha" across synapses, improving the release of glutamic acid as a memory carrier. It is produced in large batches whenever the immune system sends out an alarm for any kind of defensive action. It helps control blood clotting and is, therefore, valuable in the regulation of blood vessel flexibility. This means the healthy presence of nitric oxide in the brain may help prevent strokes.

HIGH STRESS LEVELS

John would never admit it, but he would rather have anyone else's life but his own. On the surface, this fifty-six-year-old banking executive appears to have it all. He earns a tremendous salary, travels all over the world, owns a chauffeur-driven limousine, and lives in a gorgeous manor in an exclusive area. Yet, John's seemingly perfect life is actually a never-ending parade of meetings, personnel conflicts, legal hearings, domestic battles, and problems with his children. He seldom gets more than five hours of sleep at night, and his typical answer to a headache is three aspirins and a scotch on the rocks. As far as proper nutrition, John and his driver always have a good laugh when he wolfs down his daily fast food meals while being driven in his limousine. But there is really nothing funny about it or his stressful life and lack of relaxation time.

When this busy executive began to experience dizzy spells and "holes" in his memory, he paid a visit to his doctor. It was obvious to the doctor how John's stressful lifestyle was eating away at his memory cells. Hans Selye, stress expert in the 1950s and 1960s, and author of *Stress and Aging*, warned that prolonged anxiety ages an organism, resulting in premature death. Today, we have a better understanding of the mechanism behind the concept.

The stress hormones adrenaline and cortisol provide a protective service by giving you the sudden power to either run away from or face up to a dangerous situation. Constant stress, however, takes a destructive toll on many areas of the body, including memory neurons. The constant presence of the adrenal hormone cortisol in the memory pathway overstimulates neurons to the point of death. Massive numbers of memory cells are destroyed as a result.

If John knew the link between stress, cortisol, too much calcium, and memory loss, he might make a conscious effort to reduce the stress in his life. And John is not alone. Many people constantly juggle two or three jobs at once, a behavior known as *multi-tasking*. For instance, are you the type who does things like regularly balance your checkbook while carrying on a conversation with your beautician as you get your hair cut? Or do you habitually talk on the phone while reading a newspaper and glancing at the TV? Are you famous for getting to the airport or train station with no time to spare, while dragging your luggage behind you as you talk on your cell phone? These are typical examples of multi-tasking behavior, which can lead to stress. Taking on one activity at a time, allowing more time to get to a destination, and learning to prioritize tasks and goals, will help you reduce stress and ultimately preserve memory.

If you have a tendency toward multi-tasking, try to plan your days better. Know in advance what you need to accomplish. The secret is to select and complete an activity in the order in which it will most help your daily plan. And try to avoid stressful confrontations with others.

BLOOD-BRAIN BARRIER DAMAGE

Blood vessels in memory tissue carry the same blood that circulates throughout the rest of the body. But thought and memory tissue inside the brain need to be protected from harmful substances that may have entered the body from the food you eat, the air you breathe, and the things you touch. This is where the blood-brain barrier, discussed at length in Chapter 1, comes into play.

The blood-brain barrier—a snugly fit double layer of cells that covers various memory centers in the cerebral lobes—regulates what can and cannot pass through it. It not only keeps poisons found in the outside world from harming neuronal memory tissue, it also regulates levels of amino acids like glutamic acid, which serve as message carriers inside neurons. Think of the blood-brain barrier as the inner armor that protects memory from harmful foreign invaders.

Unfortunately, the blood-brain barrier is not fail safe. Poor circulation, head trauma, tumors, and lesions can all harm this protective barrier. Memory researchers once believed the blood-brain barrier weakened with age. Now they are not so sure. Many suspect that harsh chemical substances in the environment, as well as a variety of consumer products, may be harming the ability of the of the blood-brain barrier to protect memory cells.

IN SUMMARY

Whatever makes a moment immortal comes to you by way of an ability to remember past learning in the present moment. Memory function is hardwired for extraordinary amounts of communication. Its good performance begins with sufficient amounts of oxygen for converting sugar into useable energy. Unless you have had a serious hemorrhage or blood clot in the brain that has caused irreparable damage to memory, there is good reason to believe your memory malfunction can be reversed. This is especially true if you take steps to restore fuel and energy levels in memory tissue. Never forget that your glass is half full, not half empty.

Now that you understand the physical basis for memory loss, the next chapter offers a look at some conventional causes.

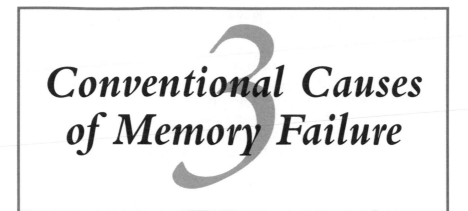

Conventional Causes
of Memory Failure

"Memory has painted this perfect day."

—Carrie Jacobs Bond

*I*t's party time and Mike spots a beautiful woman who looks very familiar. Her eye catches his as he sips his third cocktail. As she walks toward Mike, he freezes. Though she looks familiar, Mike can't remember her name or how they met. At forty-eight years old, Mike shivers at how forgetful he seems to be these days. When the woman stops to say hello, Mike, too embarrassed to admit he cannot remember her, pretends that he does, hoping that she'll give him some clue to help jog his memory. Mike's reaction is typical. When people first experience memory loss, they tend to go to great lengths to hide it.

You may not want to tell the world that you are having problems with memory failure, but the first thing you should do is communicate your problem to a neurologist who is specifically trained in memory loss. It is equally important for you to know about the well-understood, conventional causes of memory dysfunction. While many middle aged and older people have trouble remembering key details in life, memory failure is not necessarily caused by aging. Nutrient deficiency, alcohol and drug abuse, cerebrovascular disorders, electrolyte imbalance, head injury, high blood pressure, infections, tumors, and thyroid dysfunction are responsible for at least half of the memory loss cases in middle-aged adults. The good news is that most can be treated with great success.

This means you could be anywhere from forty to ninety-five years old and experience memory failure that is not due to the destructive dementia known as Alzheimer's disease. What's more, even if you *are* in the early stages of this degenerative memory robber, there is a strong probability that you can take action to curb it. In many instances, lost memory function can be brought back into a normal range if you take measures to correct the problem sooner than later.

Once you are committed to saving your memory, you must be willing to make an honest assessment of your life. Substantial changes in your living patterns and habits may become necessary. The first step is to get a thorough physical examination to determine the state of your overall health. Often, the cause of a memory complaint may be hidden behind an illness. A good exam includes tests to determine if you are a candidate for cardiovascular disease, high blood sugar, diabetes, high blood pressure, or thyroid dysfunction. Any medications that you are currently taking should be discussed with your primary health-care provider.

It is important to check the blood flow to your brain. Certain diagnostic tests can determine if blood is flowing optimally or at less than desirable levels in this area. Blood glucose levels should also be checked. Although a simple blood test can determine glucose levels, a PET scan will show how well the glucose is being converted into fuel in the brain. Blood and urine tests can ascertain levels of your important memory neurotransmitters, such as acetylcholine, norepinephrine, dopamine, glutamic acid, and glutamine.

If your doctor tells you nothing can be done about your memory dysfunction, find another doctor. Such a diagnosis is inappropriate for anyone who displays premature memory problems. Seek out another neurologist who is trained in memory loss and premature brain aging.

Because a seventy-year-old patient complained of "foggy memory with frequent confusion," his family assumed he was becoming senile. A thorough medical examination, however, indicated that the man's symptoms stemmed from an electrolyte imbalance, potassium shortage, and dehydration.

A forty-three-year-old marathon runner was mistakenly diagnosed as menopausal because her menstrual periods had stopped and her memory was on the wane. Her doctor realized that her periods had ceased because, as a runner, her body fat slipped below 12 percent. When she increased her fat ratio to 17 percent, her periods resumed, establishing that she was not menopausal. Her memory, however, continued to be poor. Only after magnesium was added in a balanced calcium supplement as part of a good vitamin and mineral program did her memory return to normal.

A fifty-four-year-old mechanic, struggling with memory dysfunction, noticed he couldn't concentrate at work because of chronic headaches. A thorough analysis by his doctor uncovered the fact that this man had hit his head during a minor skiing accident four months earlier. Even though the bump on his head had seemed minor at the time, his brain had not yet recovered totally from the injury.

These are just a few examples that show why you should not "jump the gun" and assume you have Alzheimer's disease or some other form of age-related dementia when you first experience memory loss. As you will see, there are a number of causes— causes over which you have control—that can play a part in memory loss.

NUTRIENT DEFICIENCY

The brain has always held a certain mystique, but when it comes right down to it, this two to three pound mass is made of flesh and blood. It needs to be fed just like any other tissue in the body, only more so. In fact, deficiencies of vitamins, minerals, amino acids, and enzymes can take a heavy toll on the brain's ability to process memory, fight free radical aging factors, repair brain tissue after an injury, and remove excess calcium from memory neurons.

Without the proper nutrients, the brain's delicate chemical balance is disturbed and glucose levels are lowered. Inadequate glucose prevents the energy needed to power thought and memory. When the brain is not properly fed, the oxidative "rusting" of memory cells from free radicals increases. Although some free radical damage does occur with age, proper nutrition can lessen its degenerative effects. Proper diet and supplements also help protect and preserve blood vessels, keeping them strong for normal blood circulation.

Sometimes, the right nutrients simply cannot be absorbed properly by the body. This may be the result of food allergies or improper nutrient combinations. For instance, calcium is not well absorbed without the right amount of magnesium and boron.

Where memory is concerned, poor nutrition is a fast ticket to nowhere. The good news is that you don't have to sit idly by and wait for aging to rob you of good mental function. By meeting your brain's nutritional requirements, you can extend its longevity. Be sure to turn to Chapter 6 for specific, in-depth information on a wide array of nutrients that support memory. Brain longevity—it's a very real, attainable goal.

ALCOHOL ABUSE

Howard drinks every day and forgets promises he made last week. Angered when colleagues in his law firm say he should retire, Howard still believes life is better with a glass of wine or martini in his hand. Then, there's Annette. She doesn't call a bloody Mary a cocktail, she calls it breakfast. A heavy drinker since college, Annette woke up in Manhattan the other day. She doesn't remember how she got from Miami to the Big Apple, but somehow she did.

Alcoholism affects one in every ten people who consume alcohol. A chronic condition characterized by a dependence on alcohol, chronic alcoholism eventually damages the brain, liver, and central nervous system. In terms of behavior, this condition also causes decreased mental powers, mood swings, depression, emotional outbursts, insomnia, and progressive memory loss.

As alcohol is water soluble, it passes directly from the stomach into the bloodstream. From there, the alcohol makes its way to the brain in about two to three minutes. The blood-brain barrier offers no protection and the alcohol passes through this security system with ease. Inside the brain, alcohol acts as a sensory depressant and slows the processing of information between memory neurons. Responses take longer, judgments fail, and self-monitoring is impaired. In short order, the entire nervous system is massively slowed down. Even low levels of alcohol can bring about such reactions.

Memory loss increases over time for the alcoholic. Typically, a CAT scan of the alcoholic brain shows actual shrinkage of memory tissue. Spinal fluid floods the areas that once held memory neurons.

As alcohol numbs the entire central nervous system, it erases inhibition. As their brains become more and more compromised, Howard and Annette will tend to speak unnaturally loud, make overly frank or embarrassing remarks, and never remember a word of it the next day. As long as the drinking continues, this pattern will worsen.

Visual recognition of objects is affected more by alcohol than by age. A 1997 study published in *Neuropsychology* shows that even though older people may begin to slip in memory recall ability, they still perform better than people of the same age who drink in excess.

In the early stages of alcoholism, people like Howard and Annette usually think they are very clever. They believe they are capable of focusing on whatever they want. As various memory areas are compromised, however, Howard and Annette can expect to slip into a twilight of unconcern and general disregard for themselves and others. Think of alcohol as a serious poison to memory neurons. Think of chronic, excessive drinking as a road to unfilled memories.

It is difficult to estimate just how much permanent damage has occurred in those who consume alcohol regularly. Stopping alcohol consumption will increase the chances of brain rejuvenation. Good nutrition, B-vitamin supplementation, and plenty of clean drinking water are requirements for the recovering alcoholic.

CEREBROVASCULAR DISORDERS

Carl, at age seventy-three, had been warned to get his weight down, cut out red meat, and begin an exercise regimen. He tried for a while, but wasn't motivated enough to follow through on a lifestyle change. Then one night, Carl began to feel the room spinning. He slipped to the floor as he passed out. Before the paramedics arrived, Carl—who had suffered a minor stroke—regained consciousness. He didn't remember blacking out and had no idea how long he was unconscious. Luckily, because his stroke was minor with only minimal oxygen deprivation to his brain, Carl suffered only slight memory loss. Memory loss from prolonged oxygen deprivation to neurons is very difficult, often impossible, to restore.

A disruption of blood flow to the brain means memory cells are starved for oxygen. As you saw in Chapter 2, this results in damage or death to these cells. Bleeding in or around the brain also causes damage. Disruptions that involve the brain (cerebrum) and blood vessels (vascular system), are known as cerebrovascular disorders, of which transient ischemic attacks and cardiovascular accidents, also known as strokes, are the most common.

A *transient ischemic attack* is a brief, temporary disruption in brain function caused by insufficient blood flow. It is sometimes referred to as a minor stroke. Generally the result of a temporary blockage in one of the small blood vessels leading to the brain, a transient ischemic attack is more likely to occur in those with high blood pressure, atherosclerosis, or heart disease. Though common symptoms—weakness, paralysis, or abnormal sensations on one side of the body; partial loss of vision or hearing; slurred speech; and fainting—are similar to those of a stroke, they are temporary and reversible. As these attacks are sometimes followed by strokes, their treatment is generally geared toward stroke prevention. Addressing the high risk factors for strokes, such as high blood pressure, high cholesterol, smoking, and diabetes, is often the most prudent course of action.

A *cerebrovascular accident,* more commonly known as a *stroke,* results in the death of brain tissue. Strokes are caused by lack of blood flow and insufficient oxygen to the brain. High blood pressure and atherosclerosis are the two most common causes.

There are two types of strokes: *ischemic* and *hemorrhagic.* In an ischemic stroke, blood flow to the brain is stopped due to a blocked blood vessel. This blockage is caused either by atherosclerosis or a blood clot. In a hemorrhagic stroke, a blood vessel bursts, preventing normal blood flow to the brain and causing blood leakage.

Strokes or transient ischemic attacks affect different body parts depending on the area of the brain in which the blood supply has been cut off or where the hemorrhage has occurred. For instance, blockage in the speech control area of the brain will cause slurred or impaired speech. When the brain's vision center is affected, the result can range from blurred or double vision to partial or total vision loss. Any loss of function is greatest right after a stroke. Although some of the affected brain cells may be killed, others may only be injured and eventually recover.

Despite the impairment of some brain tissue, intensive physical rehabilitation can help many people overcome the resulting disabilities of a stroke. Oxygen healing therapies, discussed in Chapter 8, can be of great assistance. In some cases, unaffected parts of the brain can take over tasks once performed by the damaged areas.

DEPRESSION

Mort, a seventy-year-old widower, appeared to be in good physical health. But he was experiencing profound memory loss, disruptive sleep patterns, and the inability to concentrate for very long. Mort's doctor first suspected the onset of Alzheimer's disease, but after thorough investigation, he discovered that Mort had recently experienced a number of upsetting incidents in his life. There was the recent death of his wife, some unexpected financial difficulties, and the relocation of his closest friend to another state. Mort was in a state of depression.

First, the doctor prescribed an antidepressant for Mort, but his memory did not improve. Further testing indicated that Mort had low levels of the neurotransmitter norepinephrine, as well as a trace mineral electrolyte imbalance—his copper levels were too high and his zinc and folic acid levels too low. Once steps were taken to correct these deficiencies and imbalances, and Mort relocated to be closer to relatives, his memory returned to normal.

Depression is commonly symptomized by long periods of intense sadness, often accompanied by a short attention span, mood swings, lack of energy, a feeling of hopelessness, obsession over the negative aspects of life, personality change, emotional fatigue, and erratic sleep patterns. Although the causes of depression are not fully understood, a variety of factors are believed to trigger its onset. Side effects from certain medications, predisposition through heredity, and emotionally upsetting events are typical causes. Biological factors such as hormonal changes, abnormal thyroid function, electrolyte imbalances, and neurotransmitter shortages are others. In some cases, depression arises for no apparent reason.

While it is true that depression and memory loss often go hand in hand, depression is not necessarily the cause of memory failure. It can, however, indicate that neurotransmitters are imbalanced and have affected the electrical charges of neurons. Studies in the 1950s at the Bio Brain Center in Princeton, New Jersey, established that trace mineral shortages or excesses play a significant role in depression. Did Mort's stress over conditions in his life drain him of neurotransmitters? Or did the lowered levels of these memory carriers make it difficult for him to respond to stress? These are burning questions for neurologists.

Unfortunately, clinical depression is a handy diagnosis when a cause cannot be established from the patient's medical history. Far too often, antidepressant drugs are prescribed because common symptoms seem to indicate depression. Yet, if a patient does not respond to an antidepressant, there's a strong possibility that he or she has been misdiagnosed. Mort was fortunate in that he was treated for the cause of his memory loss and not the symptoms.

DRUG ABUSE

Hal never got over the "highs" he enjoyed from sniffing glue in junior high. By the time he was in high school, Hal began growing his own marijuana. Soon "Happy Hal" was supplying his friends (and himself) with all the "weed" they wanted. The marijuana business was so lucrative, it enabled Hal to put himself through college. After college, Hal found himself working on Wall Street, caught up in the competitive world of stocks and bonds. Cocaine helped him grab that "extra edge" he needed in the workplace. Hal was, in the mantra of his time, "Master of the Universe." Of course, he was always so hopped up, he often needed barbiturates to sleep. By the time Hal was thirty years old, his romance with recreational drugs and sleeping potions had gotten the best of his memory. He could no longer function in his job or his personal life. Soon, he was "Master of Nowhere."

Commonly, drug abuse refers to the recreational use of illegal drugs, or the use or overuse of prescription drugs to relieve symptoms in ways not prescribed by a doctor. Alcohol, cocaine, marijuana, barbiturates, amphetamines, heroin and other narcotics, and LSD are commonly abused drugs. Often, these drugs are taken to alter the brain's function to bring about a sense of pleasure, to alleviate anxiety, or to elevate moods. And while these so-called pleasurable feelings may occur initially, continued use eventually manifests the dark side of drugs. Along with likely addiction, drug abuse is often characterized by mood swings, dizziness, unrealistic euphoria, stupor, headaches, sleep disturbances, dizziness, and failing memory.

Studies have shown that cocaine and other street drugs overstimulate certain neuron receptors in the brain's memory tissue to the point of "burnout," often to the point of no return. Just like other excitotoxins, recreational drugs destroy memory receptors. Free radical damage to brain tissue is also increased, as well as the danger of cerebrovascular and cardiovascular problems.

Prescription drugs should also be taken with great care, and only under the watchful eye of a qualified health-care professional. It is also recommended that they be taken for short periods of time to avoid possible neurotoxic effects. Even anesthesia must be used with caution—after all, these drugs are designed to erase the awareness and memory of pain during surgical procedures. If you are to undergo a surgical procedure that involves anesthesia, find out the name of the drug your surgeon is planning to use, then do some research on it. Try to discover the drug's possible side effects or cautions. Try to limit your exposure to any potential neurotoxin during your lifetime for the greatest protection of the brain and its memory.

ELECTROLYTE IMBALANCE

Biologists believe life started in ocean waters. When early life forms shifted to dry land, they evolved into animals that required extensive amounts of fluid in their bodies to fulfill chemical reactions. Even now, millions of years later, human cells still require large numbers of certain minerals known as electrolytes to regulate the electric charge and flow of molecules across the cell membrane. Electrolytes include minerals such as sodium, potassium, magnesium, calcium, carbonate, and chloride. These minerals are needed to control neuron stimulation as well as to conduct electrical impulses through nerve fibers. Crucial for memory function is the blood's electrolyte concentration, which bathes and surrounds neuron body fibers, dendrites, and axons. The electricity in the healthy brain has enough power to light a twenty-five-watt bulb.

Symptoms of electrolyte imbalance include dizziness, physical weakness, sudden onset of short-term memory loss, mental confusion, and inability to concentrate on mental tasks. Commonly, older people who are exposed to hot, dry weather or who take medicines such as laxatives, which wash electrolytes out of the body, sometimes develop low-salt levels and slip into a state of mental confusion. Such people need to guard against mineral imbalance. Always take a multimineral supplement when using laxatives. Those who consume a lot of alcohol should take a well-balanced multimineral as well. Fifty percent of the food consumed by anyone over thirty-five years old should be raw, thus abundant in life-giving, memory-protecting enzymes. (*See* The Importance of Enzymes, beginning on page 104.)

HEAD INJURY

Although the brain is protected by the thick hard bones of the skull and a cushion of spinal fluid, it is still susceptible to injury due to head trauma, also known as *traumatic brain injury*. Generally, these injuries are the result of car accidents, falls, assaults, physical abuse, and sports-related accidents. Closed-head and open-head injuries are the two types of traumatic brain injuries. In an open-head injury, the skull is penetrated, such as from a gunshot wound. In a closed-head injury, the skull is not penetrated, but the brain is injured from an external force that causes the brain to move inside the skull. A sudden jolt or blow to the head, for instance, can cause the brain to slam against the inside of the skull, damaging nerve cells and blood vessels.

Depending on the location of the injury and its severity, a brain injury can be temporary or permanent. Symptoms can include extreme or mild memory impairment, difficulty with planning and organizing, and a general decline in mental capabilities. Trauma to the skull and brain can also cause varying degrees of amnesia, or memory loss.

A head injury can sometimes trigger an inappropriate release of an antidiuretic hormone from the pituitary gland. This hormone pulls sodium from the body. Low sodium near or in the fluid surrounding neurons or the neuron fibers themselves can impact normal memory and sometimes bring on epileptic seizures in those prone to convulsions. There is always the danger of memory loss with such types of disruptions in normal nerve cell function.

HIGH BLOOD PRESSURE (HYPERTENSION)

When blood vessels become rigid, they tend to constrict and narrow. This limits blood flow and causes abnormally high pressure in the arteries, increasing the risk of strokes, aneurysms, and kidney and heart problems. In the brain, high blood pressure, also called *hypertension*, interferes with the blood flow to neurons and the memory pathways. Since nowhere is blood needed more than in the nerve cells controlling thought and memory, high blood pressure is a threat to not only memory, but to overall brain function.

Hypertension is commonly referred to as the "silent killer" because it usually causes no symptoms until complications develop. Warning signs may include shortness of breath, rapid pulse, lightheadedness, headaches, forgetfulness, and irritability.

Blood pressure is generally divided into two categories, *primary* and *secondary*. High blood pressure that is not due to another disease is considered primary hypertension and occurs in the majority of cases—about 90 percent. Although its exact cause is not known, a number of high risk factors for primary hypertension have been identified. These include stress, cigarette smoking, obesity, the excessive use of stimulants such as coffee or tea, drug and alcohol abuse, high sodium intake, and the use of oral contraceptives. Secondary hypertension, which accounts for about 10 percent of all cases, is caused by an underlying health problem, such as atherosclerosis. A buildup of fatty deposits in the arteries, atherosclerosis is the most common cause of arteriosclerosis—a thickening and hardening of the arteries. Other causes of secondary hypertension include kidney disease and hormonal disorders.

A physician will use a *sphygmomanometer* to measure blood pressure, which is represented as a pair of numbers. The first number is the *systolic* pressure; this indicates the pressure exerted by the blood when the heart beats. It signifies blood pressure at its highest. The second number is the *diastolic* pressure, which is taken between heartbeats, when blood pressure is at its lowest. Both figures represent in millimeters the height that a column of mercury reaches under the pressure exerted by the blood. For instance, a normal blood pressure reading would be 120 (systolic pressure) over 80 (diastolic pressure), and would be expressed as 120 over 80 (120/80). For adults, normal blood pressure readings range from 110/170 to 140/90. Readings of 140/90 to 160/95 indicate possible hypertension. Any pressure over 180/115 indicates severely elevated blood pressure levels. Since one blood pressure reading in a doctor's office is not conclusive, at least three readings should be taken throughout the day over two or three days.

High levels of the enzyme MAO (monamine oxidase) are associated with degenerative conditions such as dementia, depression, cerebrovascular disease, and neuritis. Until age thirty-five, MAO levels stay fairly constant and are relatively harmless. After that, MAO levels increase dramatically. Since the greatest concentration of this enzyme shows up in the brain, it makes good sense to keep its levels as low as possible. People taking MAO inhibitors, however, must be especially careful not to consume foods such as red wine, certain cheeses, and herring, which contain tyramine. Also, they should avoid the amino acid tyrosine. Such a combination might cause a stroke.

High blood pressure is particularly devastating to delicate memory nerve cells in the brain. Since an estimated 40 million men and women in the United States suffer from this condition, it is no wonder that heart attacks and strokes are the first and third leading killers in this country.

INFECTIONS

Various inflammatory viral and bacterial infections can affect the brain and destroy the environment for good memory. The human immunodeficiency virus (HIV), the herpes simplex virus, and other viruses can cause encephalitis, which can have devastating effects on the brain.

Encephalitis is an inflammation of the brain. Different types of encephalitis can either directly infect the brain and/or spinal cord, or cause an immune reaction that results in inflammation of these areas. Encephalitis can result following an outbreak of the mumps, chicken pox, or rubella. It is often characterized by symptoms such as fever, headache, vomiting, seizures, personality change, confusion, and sleepiness that can progress to a coma. Herpes encephalitis causes swelling of the brain's temporal lobe, resulting in severe brain damage. The good news is that most people with viral brain infections, including herpes encephalitis, can recover if diagnosed and treated early enough (before coma).

HIV infection—the precursor to AIDS—creates a weakened immune system, often allowing the spread of various infections. Those with AIDS may experience conditions in which specific cancers or tumors may invade the brain. Brain infections, lesions, or tumors cause dementia, memory loss, the inability to concentrate, and reduced speed of information processing.

There was a time when a major cause of memory loss and dementia stemmed from syphilis—a sexually transmitted bacterial infection. Thanks to the discovery of penicillin, this and many other bacterial infections are no longer threats. Brain dysfunction can, however, be caused by an untreated brain abscess—a localized collection of pus in the brain. A brain abscess may stem from a tooth, nose, or ear infection, from a head wound that penetrates the brain, or from an infection elsewhere in the body that is carried to the brain by the blood. Unless treated with antibiotics, a brain abscess can be fatal.

HYPOTHYROIDISM

Unkempt and sluggish, forty-nine-year-old Helen, a schoolteacher, stares blankly at a wall. She is unable to remember the name of one of her students after several minutes. Ben, a retired barber at eighty-six years old, faints in a sauna. When he regains consciousness, his words are slurred and his reaction time is slow. Once a successful carpenter, Tony, at age fifty-six, can't concentrate and has trouble learning new things.

What do all these people have in common? Each one has hypothyroidism, a condition in which an insufficient amount of thyroid hormone is produced. Because of their mental deterioration and memory loss, each feared Alzheimer's disease to be the cause. After complete physical examinations, proper thyroid supplementation was prescribed, resulting in the improvement of memory and other symptoms of each of these people.

Hypothyroidism characteristically includes a general slowing down of bodily functions. Specific symptoms include weight gain, constipation, thinning hair (particularly in women), dry skin, weak nails, anxiety, mental confusion, forgetfulness, and memory loss. The body temperature constantly runs below the normal 98.6°F.

Initially, the effects of an underactive or overactive thyroid (hyperthyroidism) are so subtle that clinicians can easily miss it. When endocrine hormones are out of balance or in the wrong proportions, brain metabolism is disrupted. This causes confusion in the neurotransmitters—the chemical message carriers of memory.

As endocrine functions begin to wane with age, it is important to get your thyroid checked after age forty, especially if you begin to suffer unexplained depression. Though women tend to develop thyroid problems more often than men, men should also be prudent about getting their thyroids checked.

IN SUMMARY

Far too often, victims of memory failure run the risk of receiving a faulty diagnosis. Many are simply told that they are suffering from depression and should be taking "happy pills," while others with more severe symptoms, especially those over age sixty, are often misdiagnosed with the onset of Alzheimer's disease.

As seen in this chapter, as well as Chapter 2, there are a number of physical and mental factors that can contribute to memory loss. And most important, most of these causes are treatable. In the next chapter, we will be making a sharp turn into some subtle, unsuspected, but equally important reasons why memory fails.

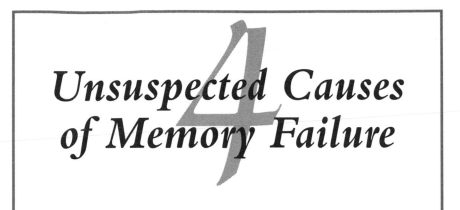

Unsuspected Causes
of Memory Failure

*"We cannot prevent the birds of sorrow from flying
over our heads, but we can refuse to let them
build their nests in our hair."*

—Chinese Proverb

Few people see the hidden, unconventional dangers of good memory from destructive forces in everyday life. Most do not understand how the toxic metals in dental fillings, cosmetics, and deodorants can inflame memory tissue. Nor do they realize the neurotoxic dangers of some commonly used food additives. And few know the dangers of the toxic chemicals found in pesticides.

Most people accept the petrochemicals, glues, and solvents used in consumer goods as safe because such items are for sale on store shelves. Few carpenters worry about the neurological risk of urea formaldehyde in building materials and pressed-wood furniture. Auto mechanics think nothing of the petrochemicals that cover their hands and clothes. And hairdressers seldom give the lead in hair dyes or the toluene in nail polish, which are absorbed into the body, a second thought. It is even harder for the public to comprehend how the invisible electromagnetic fields emitted from sewing machines, computer monitors, televisions, and electric clock radios can be bad for the delicate circuitry of memory cells.

The general public sees little connection between such items and a loss of short-term memory. It is easier to simply ignore early memory loss or accept it as a normal part of aging. But growing scientific evidence links these everyday life risks with premature memory loss. These pirates of good memory are discussed in this chapter.

EVERYDAY MEMORY PIRATES

Let's take a peek into the first hours of a typical day for Jill and Dirk. On the surface, their lives seem safe and normal. But hidden away in their daily routines are some serious threats to nerve function and memory. Using a highlighter, see how many hidden memory risks you can find.

> *The alarm on Dirk's clock radio goes off. He groans and reaches over to turn it off. Groggy, Jill struggles to find the off switch on the electric blanket. She gets up and tries to put on her slippers, but her feet are swollen. Too much wine last night, she guesses.*
>
> *Dirk rolls out of bed with another grunt. His shoulders ache, but a nice buffered aspirin and his usual ten-minute shower will take care of that. Dirk tells Jill to eat breakfast without him. The boys are getting together at that little restaurant with the bottomless coffee pot and the world's best bran muffins.*
>
> *Heading toward the kitchen, Jill enjoys the thick pile of the new carpet under her bare feet as she gathers up newspapers from the living room. She glances out the window. The orange sky signals another smoggy day. Jill makes a mental note to have more coolant added to the Bronco's radiator. Air conditioning is a definite yes today.*
>
> *Once in the kitchen, Jill turns on the TV to watch the news and draws some tap water for coffee. She squeezes fresh orange juice using the aluminum juicer she got last year in Mexico. Holding her cellular phone between her chin and shoulder, Jill makes an appointment at the hairdresser's to have her hair permed on Saturday. She then prepares a sandwich for her lunch, using that special low-fat tofu spread she got at the health food store. As she wraps the sandwich in aluminum foil, she thinks about an article she read that stated eating soy products can help prevent breast cancer. Jill adds a diet soda to her lunch bag, along with a generous assortment of chopped veggies. The people at work kid Jill about being a "health nut."*
>
> *Meanwhile, singing away in the shower, Dirk washes out the hair coloring he had applied around his hairline before shaving a few minutes earlier. He lathers up, rinses, and dries off in five min-*

utes. Dirk realizes that he hasn't been "regular" lately, so he takes a laxative. Next, he dabs on some great-smelling cologne and applies a generous amount of deodorant, as the weather report predicts the day's temperature to hit 95°F. As he starts to dress, he removes the plastic bag from a suit that has just come back from the dry cleaners. The garment's lightweight, synthetic fabric is perfect for the kind of hot day he'll be facing. At that moment, Dirk spots what looks like a flying ant on the wall. As they have had problems with termites in the past, Dirk squashes the bug and dials the exterminator on the spot.

Before heading to work, Jill plugs in her electric calculator and balances the latest entries in her checkbook. Pushing the small black box on the calculator's cord to one side with her foot, Jill glances over at her calendar and remembers that she has an appointment for a root canal later that day. Just then, a little bell dings on the microwave, signaling that Jill's frozen waffles are ready. She decides to stand and eat her breakfast while starting to get dinner ready for that evening. As Dirk is a "meat and potatoes" guy, Jill prepares meat for dinner at least three times a week. Jill pulls out an aluminum Dutch oven to which she adds a rump roast that will be slow-cooked through the day. Rushing into the bathroom, Jill takes a quick shower, then applies her deodorant and makeup, and reglues an acrylic nail that has fallen off. She looks into the mirror and admires the new, vibrant shade of lipstick she just applied. Since it is going to be a hot day, Jill slips into a dress made of a light, swishy fabric. She rushes back into the kitchen to say good-bye to her husband who is just about ready to leave.

Dirk has his laptop computer under one arm, while cradling the cell phone on his shoulder. He's speaking to the exterminating company. When he hangs up, he informs Jill that the exterminators will be out on Thursday and may have to "bag" the house. This means they'll have to go to a motel for a few days. With a kiss, Dirk flies out the door and reminds Jill to set the burglar alarm and lower the air conditioning before she leaves for work.

Dirk makes a second cellular call as he waits for the electric garage door to open. It's important for Dirk to get a jump-start on his day (he will have made at least five calls by 8:00 AM). Springing into his computerized van with its new steel-belted tires, Dirk shoots out the driveway. Looking in the rearview mirror, he wipes off Jill's lipstick and smiles. Dirk loves his life and wouldn't change a thing.

Though their lives seem safe, neither Jill nor Dirk are aware of the neurological burden placed on their bodies by the unsuspected dangers right in their own home. And don't forget, more biological land mines await them once they leave home.

Were you able to find at least forty potential factors for memory loss in the first hours of this couple's day? You did? Great! You are already aware of how to protect the neurons in your brain. If not, don't worry. Most people are unable to spot more than ten. This chapter is designed to make you aware of the unsuspected neurotoxic memory destroyers that we face every day. It's important that you start taking a hard look at these dangers and avoid them whenever you can.

A LOOK AT UNSUSPECTED DANGERS

The world is a very different place now at the end of the millennium than it was at the beginning. A thousand years ago, people had to battle hunger, bacterial infections, and other people for survival. Today, many enemies that threaten our lives are very subtle. Flavor enhancers and other chemical additives in foods, dental fillings, pesticides used on crops and in the home, furniture made with glues and formaldehyde, cosmetics, wall paints, and even artificial nails are just a few of the common items that carry threats to the nervous system and memory.

Since 1965, over 4 million synthetic compounds have been developed for consumer benefit. More than 70,000 chemical substances are commonly used in industrial manufacturing. The Environmental Protection Agency (EPA) says 30,000 of these substances were brought to the marketplace recently—between 1979 and 1995. Yet, government toxicology standards for consumer safety are vague. As a result, only four chemical substances were found to be unfit for human use during that time span. On top of that, more than 5,000 new chemical substances are estimated to appear each week for commercial use. The government does require a review of each new consumer substance before it is sold to the public, but the EPA claims that fewer than 50 percent of these chemical applications carry any safety data for human use or consumption.

If you want to protect or improve your memory, it is important to be aware of the many harmful substances that can harm your central nervous system. Do not think for one minute that because a food item has a pretty label, because a new home looks beautiful, or because electronic equipment was advertised in a trade journal that these items are safe to eat, live in, or work with. Develop a "buyer beware" attitude for all of the items you use or buy. Never be lulled by slick packaging or advertising into purchasing a service, medical treatment, food, or any other consumer item without first doing your detective work.

Let's take a closer look at some of the hidden dangers found in the foods, pesticides, dental amalgams, water, cosmetics, building materials, and electromagnetic fields that are a common part of our everyday lives.

Food Flavor Enhancers

The heat processing typically used for most foods and beverages robs them of much of their flavor. One solution for making these food items taste better is to add certain amino acids as flavor enhancers. Aspartic acid, L-cysteine, and glutamic acid—called *excitotoxins*—are the same brain chemicals that stimulate memory neurons. As these additives are obtained from plant sources, food manufacturers call them "natural" taste enhancers. These food additives, however, upset the brain's normal amino acid balance, putting the neurons into a constant state of stimulation. Eventually, overstimulation of the neurons causes them to burn out like the filament of a light bulb.

While the brain needs a certain amount of glutamic acid for a number of complex activities, too much on a continued basis destroys memory cells. Babies and people over forty years old are most susceptible. Neuron loss from glutamic acid has been documented in the key memory areas of lab animals. A small daily dose of this amino acid took only four days to begin wiping out memory neurons in ten-day old mice. Storage cells were destroyed in the hypothalamus, a key memory area that is not protected by the blood-brain barrier. The brain has it own way of naturally balancing glutamic acid, but when large amounts of it are present in the daily diet over a period of years, the brain chemistry is thrown off, setting the stage for the neuronal loss. Brain inflammation and energy loss are believed to rage out of control, resulting in memory failure.

Symptoms of damage to the brain caused by flavor enhancers include recurring headaches including migraines, attention deficient disorder, and rapid mood swings. There may be an inability to focus and complete projects as damage increases. In some cases, severe memory loss, such as the type associated with Alzheimer's, Parkinson's, and other neurological diseases, can occur.

It is often difficult to spot flavor enhancers because food manufacturers have secured what is known as "proprietary rights" in the way they describe and label ingredients on foods and drinks. Since 1984, it has been legal to hide excitotoxins under terms like "natural seasoning," "natural flavoring," "herbs," and "spices." In fact, according to current FDA regulations, the dietary additives aspartic acid and L-cysteine are not required to appear on food labels at all (see inset on page 67). With such labeling practices, consumers simply cannot tell which taste enhancers are used or in what amounts. Generally, whenever you see these terms on food labels, you can be sure the product contains flavor enhancers that will stimulate your brain to achieve artificial taste satisfaction. That pleasure is probably one of the most harmful things for memory.

The diet soda Jill packed for lunch gets its sweet taste from aspartic acid (aspartame) or Nutrasweet. The seasoned salt she put on her scrambled eggs at breakfast is loaded with glutamic acid or monosodium glutamate (MSG), and labeled as "natural flavoring." When Dirk takes a client out for lunch, which he does often, he generally goes to his favorite seafood restaurant. There, he orders his usual shrimp scampi, which has been dusted with "natural seasoning." This may be why Dirk has headaches and needs aspirin so much of the time. The effect of MSG, L-cysteine, and aspartic acid is like turning the volume up too high on a stereo speaker. Memory neurons are stimulated beyond their capacity, then they disintegrate.

It is easy enough to protect your memory from these harmful food additives. For one thing, make it your business to read food and beverage labels and watch out for the terms mentioned above. Better yet, eat more foods that are close to their natural state—ones that are locally grown and freshly picked—whenever possible.

Pesticides

Because humans are plagued with pesky bugs as well as unwanted molds and fungus infestations on plants, a wide category of chemicals have been developed to check the overgrowth of such pests. We call such chemicals pesticides, which is a broad term that covers insecticides, herbicides, and fungicides.

Pesticides work by blocking the action of specific enzymes that control life processes within an insect, plant, or fungus. The problem is that humans are exposed to these toxic chemicals, which can be inhaled or ingested. The effects of these chemicals on humans is serious. The toxins can either depress or block the flow of acetylcholine, the main message carrier in memory cells. While pesticide levels may be low and seemingly harmless, know that they are stored in body fat and accumulate over time. Here, they create

Disguising Food Flavor Enhancers

Although the FDA does not require the presence of aspartic acid and L-cysteine to appear on food labels, they do require it of glutamic acid—the major component of monosodium glutamate (MSG). Manufacturers of processed foods often use misleading ingredient names on food labels to disguise this excitotoxin. The following is a partial listing of some commonly used product names for glutamic acid.

Additives That Always Contain Glutamic Acid (MSG)

Autolyzed yeast
Calcium caseinate
Hydrolyzed protein
Hydrolyzed oat flour
Hydrolyzed plant protein
Hydrolyzed vegetable protein

Monosodium glutamate
Plant protein extract
Sodium caseinate
Textured Protein
Yeast extract

Additives That Often Contain Glutamic Acid (MSG)

Bouillon
Broth
Flavoring
Malt extract
Malt flavoring

Natural beef flavoring
Natural chicken flavoring
Natural flavoring
Seasoning
Spices

Additives That May Contain Glutamic Acid (MSG)

Carrageenan
Enzymes
Soy protein concentrate

Soy protein isolate
Whey protein concentrate

inflammation and damaging changes to the genetic code of body cells. Although the liver's job is to filter poisons out of the body, it is able to filter only those poisons that are water soluble, not those that are fat-soluble.

Since the myelin sheath that protects the brain's neurons is made up of fat, scientists believe toxins from pesticides are likely to be stored there. This helps contribute to neuron inflammation due to allergic responses—the body's own attempt to protect you from foreign substances. Such "fire" in the brain is associated with memory loss.

Remember, since the liver cannot filter pesticides from the body fat, these chemicals accumulate throughout your life. This is another reason it is important to reduce dietary fat intake. The less fat you have, the less storage for pesticides and other toxins.

Symptoms of pesticide poisoning are difficult to pin down because of the poison's low-level exposure pattern. In other words, the toxicity builds gradually over time. Of course, sudden exposure to high pesticide levels can have immediate reactions that can range from flu-like symptoms that commonly include wheezing and general respiratory problems, to convulsions, paralysis, and even coma. Other eventual symptoms may include failing memory, unexplained personality changes, and irritability. Both men and women can experience reduced fertility. For some reason, the body relates to a pesticide the way it does to estrogen. Women with high levels of pesticide toxins often experience hot flashes and the discomfort of premenstrual syndrome. Both sexes are believed to experience more frequent viral infections as well as serious immune problems that can lead to food allergies, arthritis, chronic fatigue syndrome, premature aging, and certain skin problems.

Pesticides Used for Pest Control

It is alarming that our friend Dirk immediately called the exterminator to come out and possibly "bag" the house. Many commercial insecticides used by exterminators can stay active in a home for up to twenty years. This means that Jill and Dirk's memory tissue will be under constant exposure to neurotoxins through breathing and skin contact. Like Jill and Dirk, most people have no idea of the danger to which they are exposing their memory tissue when they allow insecticides to be applied inside the home.

Common household insecticides like diazinon, malathion, dursban, and lindane are linked to brain and memory diseases as well as psychological problems, including depression. Pesticides have also been linked to physical motor problems. Often, people with even moderate levels of these chemicals will show a diminished ability to think and process memory. Spontaneous mood swings, unexplained anger, and unreasonable anxiety are other results from such neurotoxins. Yet, it is very hard to track such a problem because in many instances the toxins build up over time. Scientists have learned of these physical and mental responses through patterns established in large field studies or from experimental research in the laboratory.

Pesticides and Foods

Pesticides ingested in the foods we eat are an even more serious problem than those used for home pest control. Unless the veggies Jill likes to eat are organically grown without the use of pesticides, they have been grown in a conventional manner. This means they have been sprayed with insecticides, herbicides, and/or fungicides. So if Jill and Dirk aren't breathing the neurotoxic substances, they are eating them in the very fruits and vegetables they believe to be healthy.

In 1962, Rachel Carson warned of the dangers of pesticides like the now-banned DDT in her classic work *Silent Spring*. At that time, an estimated 300 million pounds of pesticides were used on crops grown in the United States. Today, that number has grown to over 800 million. People may think that pesticides affect only molds, fungi, and insects, but they're wrong. More than 338,000 cases of human reactions to toxic pesticide exposure were recorded between 1985 and 1990 in the United States. Various insecticides, fungicides, herbicides, and rodenticides were found to be the cause of 63 percent of the deaths from toxic exposure reported at poison control centers during that time period.

Worldwide, the pesticide poisoning problem is even greater. The World Health Organization (WHO) estimates that 3 million cases of severe pesticide poisoning occur each year outside the United States. In developing nations, 25 million farm workers suffer from pesticide-related poisoning at least once a year. U.S. Customs records show that we are shipping pesticides that are banned here to countries overseas at the rate of 2.5 tons per hour!

This is of special concern because these very pesticides are used on grains, fruits, and vegetables that are grown abroad, particularly in South America. These products are then shipped back to the United States for sale in our local supermarkets. And think about this, only one in approximately every hundred trucks transporting produce across the Mexican border will be checked for acceptable pesticide levels. And even then, just one or two pieces of produce are checked.

How to Cope With Pesticides

There are a number of things you can do to lower your risk of exposure to toxins from common household pesticides, as well as those found in foods. When it comes to food, simply be careful in choosing what you eat. Whenever possible, opt for produce that has been organically grown and pesticide-free. You might even consider starting your own backyard garden. If you buy commercially grown leafy vegetables, always remove and discard the outer leaves, which often contain greater amounts of pesticides than the inner leaves. Wash all commercially grown produce well with warm water and a little liquid detergent. This will remove up to half the surface pesticide residue. Be sure to scrub or peel fruits and vegetables, especially root varieties. And avoid imported produce, which may have been treated with banned or unregulated chemicals.

There are a variety of ways to lower your risks from the dangerous toxins found in commonly used household and yard pesticides. First of all, always opt for nontoxic alternatives first. For instance, try getting rid of ants by spraying them with mint tea. Sprinkling borax or chili powder at the site where ants are entering your home will keep them from coming in. Plant mint around the foundation of your house; it is a natural insect repellent. When fighting subterranean colonies of termites, investigate the possibility of using nematodes—microscopic worms that secrete a bacteria that kills insects such as termites so they can eat them. Nontoxic to humans, nematodes are available at many garden supply stores. Another nontoxic alternative for termite control is a special soap called timbor, which is forced by machine into termite colonies, where it eventually destroys the pests. Timbor is available from the United States Borax Company (300 Falcon Street, Wilmington, CA 90744; 1–310–522–5300). Dry-wood termites can be killed by heating the infested area to 140°F for a short period of time.

And let's not forget about insect repellents, many of which contain harmful chemicals like DEET (N, N-diethyl-m-toluamide). These are especially harmful if applied directly to the skin. Instead, try one of the many natural, nontoxic insect repellents on the market today, such as *Skin So Soft* by Avon Products (9 West 57th Street, New York, NY 10019; 1–800–858–8000), *Beat It!* by Naturpath (1410 NW 13th Street, Gainesville, FL 32601; 1–800–542–4784), and *EcoZone Skeeter Shoo* by Natural Animal Health Products, Inc. (PO Box 1177, St. Augustine, FL 32085; 1–800–274–7387).

If you have any questions regarding the risks or benefits of specific pesticides, call the National Pesticides Telecommunications Network at 1–800–858–PEST. For information on nontoxic alternatives for pest control contact the Bio-Integral Resource Center (BIRC), Box 7414, Berkeley, CA 94707 (1–510–524–2567). The books *Safe Shopper Bible* by David Steinman and Samuel Epstein (New York: MacMillan Publishing, 1995), *Bug Busters* by Bernice Lifton (Garden City Park, NY: Avery Publishing Group, 1991), and *Pest Control You Can Live With* by Debra Graff (Sterling Heights, VA: Earth Stewardship Press, 1990) are excellent sources of nontoxic pest control suggestions.

Heavy Metals

Certain metals in nature have a molecular weight that is at least five times that of water. One exception is aluminum, but since this metal is found in large amounts in the neuronal tissue of Alzheimer's victims, we have included it along with arsenic, cadmium, lead, and nickel as a hazard for memory function. When these heavy metals get into the brain, they create havoc on memory function by increasing neuron tissue permeability. This means important nutrients necessary for brain function actually flow out of the very tissue that needs them. When this happens, the chemistry of the neuron's dendrites and axons, as well as the synaptic gap between neurons is thrown off balance. Neurotransmitter production is endangered, slowing down the speed of information input.

Symptoms of heavy metal contamination in the body include poor memory, inability to focus for long on a topic, chronic low body temperature, constipation on a regular basis, facial ticks, shaking hands or feet, unusual skin blistering or rashes, and joint or limb deformity.

Under normal circumstances, your body produces antioxidant enzymes—vacuum-cleaner like substances that neutralize harmful waste into water and ordinary oxygen. Such waste materials are called free radicals because they are the lone, unstable electrons looking to form a stable bond. Think of free radicals as broken glass on your kitchen floor. If you sweep it up before someone steps on it, no harm will be done. Antioxidant enzymes are able to provide the extra electron that neutralizes waste in the body, allowing it, like the glass on your kitchen floor, to be swept out of the body as plain water and harmless oxygen. Heavy metals interfere with the production of these important garbage-collecting antioxidant enzymes. They also put memory neurons at a disadvantage by damaging their protective blood-brain barrier.

Aluminum

Although aluminum is not a heavy metal, it can be toxic if it is deposited in the brain. Typically, during autopsies of Alzheimer's patients, aluminum has been found in large amounts in the neuronal tissue. This accumulation of aluminum in the brain has been implicated in seizures and reduced mental function. Although elemental aluminum is not able to pass through the blood-brain barrier easily, certain aluminum compounds such as aluminum fluoride can.

The average person takes in between 3 and 10 milligrams of aluminum every day, absorbed primarily through the digestive tract, but also through the lungs and skin. Because aluminum is present in the air, water, and soil, it is found naturally in food and water. It is also found in cookware, cooking utensils, and foil. Many other products contain aluminum as well, including deodorant, baking powder, antacids, table salt, some laxatives, toothpaste, and construction materials. The exhaust fumes from cars with aluminum engines is another source.

Arsenic

Traces of arsenic are found in pesticides, laundry detergents, car exhaust fumes, additives fed to livestock, smog, tobacco smoke, and table salt. Accumulation of this heavy metal is associated with blinding headaches, drowsiness, and confusion. Chronic arsenic poisoning can result in certain types of cancer, coma, and even death.

Cadmium

Like lead, cadmium accumulates in the body and has varying degrees of toxicity. Besides creating mental and physical fatigue, cadmium damages neurons in the spinal column. It can also lead to breathing problems, which limit oxygen flow to memory neurons. Excessive amounts lead to high blood pressure. Collecting in the kidneys, cadmium is also associated with kidney stones.

Cigarette smokers as well as those exposed to second-hand smoke often have high levels of cadmium in their bodies. Cadmium is also found in increased amounts in plastics and in the production of nickel-cadmium batteries. Other common sources of cadmium include silver polish (always wear gloves when using it), pesticides, and refined grains.

Lead

Highly toxic, lead is one of the most widely used metals today. Exposure can lead to depression, vertigo, irritability, headaches, confusion, and lowered IQ. Lead poisoning can lead to paralysis, blindness, and mental disturbances including memory loss. Chronic lead poisoning can lead to reproduction disorders, impotence, coma, and even death. Even low-levels of lead accumulation in young children have been associated with impaired intellectual development and/or temporary or permanent brain damage.

Sources of lead exposure include lead-based paints, ceramic glazes, lead crystal glassware, leaded gasoline, tobacco, lead-soldered cans, pesticides, and auto exhaust fumes. Cow's milk can be contaminated with lead if the animal was fed fodder that contained lead. Water that flows through lead piping—used in most homes built before 1930—is another source. Although newer homes use copper pipes, many of these pipes are soldered with lead, which can leach into the water, especially during the first few years after installation. The good news is that lead solder was banned in 1986.

Mercury

One of the most toxic metals, mercury is found in our soil, water, and food supply, as well as in pesticides. Because methyl mercury is present in our water supply, large amounts are found in fish, especially larger types that are high on the food chain. Mercury is also present in a number of common everyday products, such as cosmetics, fabric softeners, ink for printers and tattooists, solvents, and wood preservatives. Dental fillings are the biggest contributor.

Mercury is a cumulative poison. Retained in the pain center of the brain, it can prevent the entry of nutrients into the cells, as well as the removal of waste from the cells. Significant amounts can produce arthritis, depression, muscle weakness, and severe memory loss.

Over 180 million Americans have amalgam dental fillings—a major source of mercury exposure. Dental amalgams contain 50 percent mercury, 25 percent silver, and 25 percent other materials, such as copper and nickel. According to the World Health Organization, 2 to 15 micrograms of mercury are released every day from these fillings either in the form of vapors or actual chips that come off when you chew food. The mercury is either absorbed into the brain via soft tissue in the mouth, through delicate nasal tissue, or through the digestive tract.

Mercury "burden" studies throughout the industrialized world have found a link between the number of amalgam surfaces and mercury levels in memory neurons. The more amalgams you have, the more mercury will be found in sensitive areas of learning and recall. The hippocampus, as the first base for short-term memory, is especially hard hit by mercury buildup. So is the emotional memory center—the amygdala. A third area that is also affected by high mercury levels is the nucleus basalis of Meynert—an important cognitive area of memory.

The American Dental Association continues to deny that mercury is a problem when used as a dental filling. Yet, an army of medical researchers disagree. Scientific research has found that people with severe memory loss characteristic of Alzheimer's disease have higher amounts of mercury and aluminum in their brain tissue than people who do not have such memory loss. A number of people who have suffered for years from various health problems, including candidiasis, chronic fatigue, and recurrent infections, found that these problems cleared up after their amalgam dental fillings were removed.

If you choose to have your amalgam fillings replaced with less toxic porcelain or resin fillings, do not have more than two or three done at a time. Wait at least six months, if possible, between such replacements. And make certain the dentist uses a rubber dam to prevent any mercury shavings from touching, even for a second, the tissues that line your mouth. An assistant should also be present with a special suction device to clean up the mercury as soon as it is removed. Some dentists have started using oxygen masks for patients as well as themselves when removing dental amalgams.

The American Dental Association has lobbied for legislation that makes it illegal in many states for dentists to suggest that your health might improve if mercury amalgam fillings are removed. In fact, in certain areas of the country, a well-meaning dentist can lose his or her license for making such a suggestion! So you must suggest amalgam replacements yourself.

In view of the growing amount of important research showing a direct connection between Alzheimer's disease and the use of mercury amalgam fillings, it is time for the United States to join the many other nations who already ban the use of mercury in filling material.

Nickel

Although minute amounts of nickel are important in a number of body functions, too much can be toxic. Excessive amounts can cause skin rash and respiratory illness, and it can interfere with cellular energy production. Significant nickel levels can also lead to free radical damage in the brain, dim vision, poor digestion, and hoarseness.

Significant amounts of nickel are contained in tobacco smoke and hydrogenated fats that are commonly used in fast food operations. It is also found in stainless steel cookware and is leached out by acidic foods like tomato sauce. Refined and processed foods are also culprits. The main source of nickel toxicity in the body is from dental materials, such as fillings and braces. Be sure to check to see if your dentist uses materials with this alloy. Ask for nontoxic alternatives.

Contaminated Water

It's no secret that bathing and drinking water in the United States is becoming increasingly contaminated thanks to the dumping of toxic waste into rivers and landfills. Clean water is vital for good memory. Water that contains toxic metal residue, for instance, places an extra burden on the liver and kidneys—the body's main filtering units. When such metals are present in the blood, there is an increased probability of free radical damage and damage to the blood-brain barrier that protects neurons. Then there are the four areas of the brain that are not protected by the blood-brain barrier. The neurons in these unprotected locations are at the mercy of the oxidative forces of the contaminants in the water.

The skin—the body's largest organ—can absorb neurotoxins through its pores. Therefore, the water you use for your shower or bath, like the water you drink, should be clean and nontoxic. When Dirk takes his ten-minute morning shower, he is exposing himself to any number of industrial waste materials, because his city's water plant (typical of most plants) does not remove solvents, pesticides, heavy metals, or other neurotoxic substances from the water supply. Although a healthy person is absorbing neurotoxins from the water, he or she may not show any negative symptoms. But the individual with an already-depressed immune system will contribute to immune overload each time he or she bathes in contaminated water. It is vital to protect the blood-brain barrier and surrounding memory tissue from such contaminated water.

The plumbing in your house may contain pipes that are lead soldered. As the lead will leach into the water, always allow the water to run for at least thirty seconds before using it, especially if you do not have a water filter. Municipal water departments make an effort to keep city drinking water safe from harmful bacteria and viruses. Most often, however, they do not filter out heavy metals, pesticides, fungicides, or other chemicals.

Each time you move into a new house, apartment, or office, have the water analyzed. Even if a house or condo is new, don't trust the plumbing. And do not hesitate to test the water that comes from your water filter for lead.

If your local government health agencies do not perform water tests, you can order a test kit from a certified independent laboratory. Test kits provide special containers along with instructions for obtaining water samples. The samples are then returned to the laboratory for analysis. The following companies provide water-test kits: National Testing Labs, 6151 Wilson Mills Road, Cleveland, OH 44143, 1–800–458–3330; WaterTest Corporation, PO Box 186, New London, NH 03257, 1–800–426–8378; and Suburban Water Testing Labs, 4600 Kutztown Road, Temple, PA 19560, 1–800–433–6595. Depending on the test results, the companies will advise you on possible plans of action.

A home water-filtration system is strongly suggested. You can choose a system that is designed to purify your entire household water supply, or opt for a point-of-source filter system, which is less expensive. Point-of-source systems are attached to a single water source, such as a kitchen faucet, to purify cooking and drinking water, or to an individual shower head to purify water for bathing and showering. To locate companies that install water filter systems, check the yellow pages of your local telephone directory under "Water Filtration and Purification Systems."

Candidiasis and Food Allergies

Candidiasis is an infection caused by an overgrowth of the *Candida albicans* organism and other candida species, which live in the gastrointestinal tracts of healthy persons. Under normal conditions, candida lives in healthy balance with other bacteria in the body.

When candida is allowed to rocket out of control—due to such causes as the use of antibiotics or immunosuppressive drugs, or a sugar-laden diet—it can transform itself from an innocuous, rootless yeast into an aggressive and tenacious fungus. At this stage, the fungus puts down roots, which can penetrate the lining of the intestines, causing what is known as a *leaky gut*. When the intestinal walls are breached, partially digested food particles, bacteria, and other materials are able to pass directly into the bloodstream. Because these substances do not belong in the blood, the immune system is called into action to fight the invaders. This defense response increases inflammation in the blood. In turn, this inflammation is passed on to the memory neurons receiving the blood. When this happens over and over, a constant drain is placed on the immune system. Eventually, the immune system will be too weak to handle the undigested food particles and your body will become allergic to that food.

In addition, the candida toxins can integrate into the body's hormonal secretions. This can affect the brain and nervous system. Symptoms may include fatigue, apathy, loss of energy, headaches, irritability, depression, and memory lapses.

When treating candidiasis, it is important to watch your diet and avoid certain products, including antibiotics, immunosuppressive drugs, steroids, birth control pills, and cigarettes. Refined and concentrated sugar products should be avoided as well.

Intestinal Parasites

A parasite is an organism, such as a single-celled protozoan or worm, that lives in another organism called a host. Microscopic parasites can enter your body through foods you eat, beverages you drink, or items you touch.

The problem with any type of parasite is that it robs its host of valuable enzymes and nutrients, such as vitamin B_{12}, leaving behind toxic poisons in the body cells. Parasites that infect the intestines may burrow through the intestinal wall, causing a leaky gut. In the same way that was explained in the previous discussion on candidiasis, the leaky gut allows food substances and bacteria to pass through the intestine into the bloodstream. The immune system then attacks the invaders, resulting in blood inflammation. Especially in the aging brain, constant inflammation is very dangerous for memory. It places a burden on the blood-brain barrier, eventually causing neurons to overheat and die.

Symptoms of parasitic infestation include gas, nausea and vomiting, constipation or diarrhea, stomach discomfort, and abdominal bloating. Research indicates that over 7 million Americans have intestinal parasites. Possibly due to high immigrant populations and unsanitary conditions, certain cities like New York and places like Southern California have a substantial number of residents (12 to 14 percent) who are infected with parasites. Medical experts at Albert Einstein Medical School suspect as much as 20 percent of the total U.S. population at any given time is infested with intestinal parasites. *Giardia lamblia, Entamoeba histolytica,* and *Blastocystis hominis,* typically transmitted through contaminated food and water, are the most common.

The body's natural immune defenses are almost helpless in controlling these intestinal parasites because they live *inside* cells. This hiding place makes it difficult to develop vaccines against intestinal protozoa. A number of drugs and natural products are available to help rid the body of parasites. Grapefruit seed extract, for instance, is a natural alternative that is effective in killing parasites found in the digestive tract. Clearing these microscopic organisms decreases the body's immune burden.

Cosmetics and Other Image Enhancers

Comedian and actress Mae West once said you are never too old to look young. Today, most people seem to agree. Billions of dollars worldwide are spent on perfumes and colognes, makeup, skin moisturizers, after-shave lotions, hair dyes, nail-care products, hair removers, deodorants, shampoos, and hair conditioners, all to improve appearance and maintain physical appeal. Don't get the wrong idea. We're not trying to dampen your fun. We just want you to be aware of some of the ways in which these products can have a negative impact on your memory.

Cosmetics are capable of causing a number of negative reactions. For instance, a skin rash may appear after applying moisturizing lotion, fingertips may feel numb or tingly after an acrylic nail application, and a metallic taste may develop after applying hair color. Other reported reactions to makeup and cosmetics include dizziness, puffy eyes, skin rashes, confusion, mood swings, lack of concentration, and short-term memory loss. When Jill begins her morning makeup regimen, she is exposing her skin to a wide array of neurotoxic chemicals. But like most people, Jill assumes if a beauty product is on the store shelf, it's safe.

The problem is only 2 percent of the 3,400 makeup ingredients used in the early 1980s had adequate chemical analysis to ensure safety for the public. While limited information could be found for 1,400 of these ingredients, no safety data was available for more than 1,900 ingredients in a 1984 survey. Since nerve endings and blood vessels lie close to the skin's surface, it is shocking that more information about such substances is not available for a trusting public.

Although the Food and Drug Administration (FDA) is the governing agency of the cosmetic industry, it has little authority over controlling the use of harmful substances in various cosmetic products. The bottom line is that the cosmetic industry can use and sell any substance in makeup and toiletry products without government approval. They must, however, list the ingredients on the label.

Let's not forget the role of the manufacturers, who rush products to the marketplace in an effort to capture profits. And then there are the advertisers, who are so eager for new product promotion they offer no resistance. Scientific researchers tend to follow the money as well. Few study grants fund projects that determine the risks of body enhancement products. Without giving much thought to the consequences, consumers buy these products regardless of their lack of safety testing.

All sorts of neurotoxic chemicals lurk in many of the items in your beauty regime. Once absorbed through the skin or the gut lining into the blood, these poisons place an extra inflammatory burden on the hypothalamus, the center of immune function. As part of the limbic system, the hypothalamus coordinates immune defense functions throughout the body. Here, inside this tiny cluster of neurons, complex chemical decisions are made to protect you against normal invaders like viruses, bacteria, molds, and fungi.

This defense system that is housed in the brain took millions of years to evolve, but, as mentioned earlier, the hypothalamus has one glaring weakness. Like a castle without a moat, the hypothalamus lacks the protection of the blood-brain barrier to save it from neurotoxic substances such as those found in cosmetics. Without this protective two-cell layer, the hypothalamus is vulnerable to the unnatural, synthetic chemicals and heavy metals present in many cosmetic products on the market today. Many beauty products enjoy a close "intimacy" with your body. Once neurotoxic substances in cosmetics get into the blood, they can eventually contaminate nerve tissue. Free radical damage increases and eventually memory neurons die.

The hypothalamus uses various defense methods to fight the effects of neurotoxins in cosmetics. But such immune responses on a day-to-day basis create too much inflammation, which spreads to other parts of the limbic system, including the hippocampus and the amygdala. Pretty soon, neurons inside key memory areas of the limbic system burn up and disappear. When you have lost a certain percentage of nerve cells in these areas, you will start having trouble with short-term memory.

Let's now take a brief look at some of the culprits found in the commonly used beauty products used every day.

Hair-Care Products

Hair colorants, shampoos, conditioners, styling gels, and hair sprays all contain harmful chemicals. More than any other profession, hairstylists have a high incidence of allergies. This is undoubtedly because of their constant toxin absorption through fumes and skin contact from hair-care products.

Hair dyes for men are especially neurotoxic because of the lead acetate they contain. Bleaching products to lighten the hair appear to be less neurotoxic and cancer causing than brown, black, and red dyes. But hydrogen peroxide, a free radical, is added to both dyes and bleaches and is absorbed into the scalp along with other toxic chemicals such as phenylenediamine, diethanolamine (DEA), and triethanolamine (TEA), and dyes like FD&C Yellow 5 and D&C Red 33.

Since the hypothalamus helps regulate immune function, it is important to keep neurotoxic elements away from such memory tissue. Do you really want to put such caustic substances on your scalp? Your thinking cap, the cerebral cortex, lies only a short distance away.

A number of gentle color rinses and semi-permanent hair coloring products are now available. Unlike permanent hair color, these products typically contain very little peroxide and no ammonia. They are "deposit-only" hair colorants that are designed to simply coat the hair with a protein-based pigment. This helps cover gray hair to some degree, but not totally and not for very long. Men might consider using these hair coloring products themselves. Remember to always read product disclaimers with care. They warn of the possible product side effects, such as skin irritation. Safer, more natural hair colorants such as those from Logona, Rainbow Research, and Igora Botanic are sold in many health food stores. You can also try the nineteenth-century remedy of covering gray hair by combing a brew of strong black tea through it after shampooing.

Before using any shampoo, first read the ingredients on the label. Be sure DMDM hydantoin, 2-bromo-2-nitropropne-1,3-diol, and polyethylene glycol, which change into the neurotoxin formaldehyde, do not appear. Dandruff shampoos tend to be the most toxic. Ecco Bella, Desert Essence, Bindi, Logona, Nature's Gate, Urtekram, and Paul Penders are safer hair shampoo brands.

When choosing a hair conditioner, select one that does not contain quaternium 15, polysorbate 80, or formaldehyde. Aubrey, Desert Essence, Earth Science, Nature's Gate, Paul Penders, and Rainbow Research brands are less-toxic than many commercial brands. For a truly natural conditioner that works remarkably well on bleached or permed hair, try a twenty-minute mayonnaise treatment. After covering your hair with mayonnaise, tie it up with a plastic bag. Then relax in a hot tub for twenty minutes. You'll probably need two shampoos to get the mayonnaise out, but the results are worth it. A beer rinse is also an effective conditioner, if you don't mind the smell.

Hair sprays that come in aerosol cans emit neurotoxic particles that are so small they can easily be breathed into the innermost parts of your lungs. From this point, it is merely a short jump into the blood. And remember, blood circulates throughout the brain every two to three minutes. Just breathing the spray can bring on coughing and breathing difficulty for some people. Pump containers of hair sprays are less toxic, but not much. Certain sprays contain alcohol that can be tainted with toxic 1,4-dioxane. Avoid spray and gel products with padimate-O, butylated hydroxyanisole (BHA), TEA, DEA, and any of the FD&C dyes. Always cover your eyes, mouth, and nose if you use any hair spray, and be sure there is a fan or open window nearby. Less toxic hairsprays and gels are made by Aubrey, Earth Preserve, Earth Science Silk, and Alexandra Avery Hair Oil.

Makeup

It is important to be aware of the presence of aluminum lakes (pigments), which bind and hold color in many types of makeup. Lipsticks, blushes, eye shadows, and face powders typically contain aluminum lakes. Chemists representing the cosmetic industry argue that the aluminum molecules found in makeup are too large to be absorbed through cell membranes (either through the skin or the intestinal wall) and are, therefore, not dangerous. Studies conducted in Germany, however, indicate large aluminum molecules are, in fact, able to pass through the gut wall into the blood.

Also, studies funded by private sources show that women tend to have twice as much trouble with memory loss in later years than men. Although this has been attributed to drops in estrogen, also consider that women generally use more makeup than men—a possible contributing factor.

Many lipsticks contain neurotoxic coal tars, which have been implicated in headaches, mood shifts, and allergic reactions. But the biggest problem with most lipsticks is that most brands contain aluminum lakes. Once applied, lipstick is easily swallowed along with foods and beverages. The aluminum then finds its way easily into the bloodstream and on to the brain where it can invade those areas not protected by the blood-brain barrier. While the levels may be slight, over a lifetime, the cumulative damage could be significant. Just how much aluminum passes to the brain from lipstick and other cosmetics in this manner has yet to be determined. A lot of so-called "natural" lipsticks are coming to market without carcinogenic dyes, but be sure to check them for aluminum lakes. And always blot lipstick after application to minimize the amount swallowed. Safer lipstick brands include Ecco Bella, Rachel Perry, and Paul Penders.

Blush products give the face a touch of color and vibrancy. Look for blushes that do not contain BHA, formaldehyde, and/or quaternium 15. Irritants like propylene glycol and imidazolidinyl can inflame cell tissue. To be on the safe side, avoid cheek color with D&C Red and FD&C Yellow dyes. Talc is probably not harmful on the skin, but when inhaled, it can irritate the lining of your lungs. And yes, aluminum lakes are used in blushes as well. Shop for less toxic blushes such as those by Dr. Hauschka, Ecco Bella, Ida Grae, and Paul Penders.

Face powder absorbs oils and gives the face a nice refined appearance. But key ingredients in powder, such as quaternium 15 and 2-bromo-2 nitropropane, subject you to formaldehyde, a definite neurotoxin. How much do you absorb through the skin? Once again, nobody knows because it has not been well examined by nonbiased research. Our concern is based on the inflammatory tendencies of formaldehyde to harm the nervous system. While the amount of formaldehyde absorbed through face powder is probably negligible, it can be just another small "hit" against blood immune factors controlled by the hypothalamus and other parts of nerve tissue in the brain. Over a lifetime, the exposure adds up.

Do not think that expensive brands of face powders are better than cheaper ones. Pressed powders with 2-bromo-2-nitropropane-1,3-diol can go through complicated chemical changes and end up as formaldehyde, no matter what the cost. Face powder made by Bare Escentuals and Aubrey are probably the least toxic brands.

Eye shadow works for the modern woman just like it did for Cleopatra. But, again, watch out for aluminum lakes and quaternium 15, which can harm nerves in the eyes. The entire eye mechanism is just too close to nerve tissues in the brain. As with face powder, the damage occurs with repeat usage over many years. If you must wear eye shadow, try those by Beauty Without Cruelty, Bare Escentuals, Ecco Bella, Dr. Hauschka, and Paul Penders.

Deodorants and Antiperspirants

We are a nation obsessed with smelling good, as well as looking good. Many deodorants and antiperspirants, which may be effective in preventing body odor, often contain aluminum. So here we are back at the aluminum-Alzheimer's connection. In addition, many deodorants contain zirconium, which can cause underarm inflammation. The presence of magnesium and zinc oxides help curtail zirconium irritation. Due to increased body temperature under the arms, harmful substances are absorbed there more easily. And don't forget that part of the lymphatic system is located there, as well. Safer brands of deodorants include Faberge Power Stick, Desert Essence, Lady Speed Stick, Secret Roll-On, Suave Stick, and Weleda Sage. There is even an effective natural deodorant that is actually a piece of mineral salt.

Nail Care Products

Take a good look at your nails. Their job is to protect the ultra-sensitive nerve endings in your fingers. A condition known as *paresthesia* can occur when neurotoxic substances from polishes, nail glues, or solvents seep through nail tissue, causing a numbing, burning sensation in the fingertips. Artificial nails of any type and various nail polishes may make nails look nice, but not much safety data exists for the ingredients found in such products. Solvents like toluene, which are used in various nail preparations, are known neurotoxins. And let's not forget about the dangerous neurotoxic fumes from these items.

Ammonia, formaldehyde, and chloride fumes—common elements in nail products—are neurotoxic. While artificial nails and polish are not recommended, if you do apply them, be sure to do so in a well-ventilated area. This will help prevent you from inhaling any noxious fumes, which can place a burden on the blood-brain barrier. And once the blood-brain barrier, which encases precious neurons, becomes compromised, your good memory will start to fade.

The glues and acrylics used for artificial nails bring another neurotoxic concern—they tend to thin the nail surface, increasing the risk of fungal infections, which can affect neural endings in fingertips. If nails look stained or yellowed after nail polish is removed, there is a strong possibility that dyes from the polish are being absorbed into the nerve endings of your fingertips, adding a neurotoxic burden. Nail products by De Lore appear to be somewhat safe, but we strongly recommend going for the bare, natural look in nail care.

Fragrances

Have you ever walked into a department store and been sprayed with perfume? We are a nation that loves to smell good, however, more people than ever before are registering complaints, such as headaches, memory loss, mental confusion, and mood swings, in connection with perfumes and other product fragrances. One man we know had to cancel a magazine subscription because the publisher placed pull-out perfumed advertisements inside each issue. A forty-four-year-old woman developed blinding headaches and breathing difficulties after applying a new brand of deodorant. She discovered that toluene—a chemical found in the deodorant's fragrance—caused the reactions.

Adding fragrance to consumer items like soaps, skin lotions, and even cleaning products and furniture polishes is very big business in the United States. However, widespread use does not guarantee safety. Since reliable product testing is so limited, just be aware that the various substances used in the perfume trade carry neurotoxic risks for memory.

Have you noticed how many fragrances linger in the air long after the person wearing it has passed by? Or have you tried to wash perfume out of your hair or clothing, only to discover it was not an easy task? What if these chemicals adhere to nasal cells in the same way? How is your body to clean them out? What are their long-term effects on memory cells once they have penetrated brain tissue? Nobody knows.

Clean air and natural scents are the only things that should pass through the nasal passages. Oxygen molecules need to go through the lungs to be absorbed for important cell metabolism in memory tissue and elsewhere in the body. But we suspect some of the modern perfume scents are just too well targeted for excitatory areas of the brain and may actually harm brain tissue. Which parts and where we cannot say because, again, there is insufficient third-party safety research.

This section may have seemed like a splash of cold water on body image enhancement. We are not suggesting you arrive at a party looking or smelling like Godzilla's cousin. But do create some boundaries. Shop for products with minimal neurotoxic ingredients. And write to manufacturers. Let them know your desire for safe, nontoxic body-enhancement products. Demand more for your money.

Read *The Safe Shopper's Bible* by David Steinman and Samuel Epstein, MD (NewYork: MacMillan Publishing, 1995) for an extensive amount of product safety research. Hundreds of household and consumer brands have been researched and ranked for safety in easy-to-follow coded charts.

Building Materials

When Jill and Dirk were shopping for a home, they fell in love with a newly constructed house that overlooked a creek with a wide expanse of trees below. However, after being in the house for only twenty minutes, they both noticed that they had developed headaches. Because Jill and Dirk had read Raymond Singer's *Neurotoxicity Guidebook* (New York: Van Nostrand Reinhold, 1990), they were aware that their headaches were probably coming from the building materials. They thanked the realtor and decided to buy an older unit up the street.

Thousand of toxic chemicals are found in the home and workplace in such common products as carpeting, paints, kitchen counters, cabinets, and glues. While the emission of noxious fumes, called *off-gassing*, from an individual source may not be a risk in itself, most homes have many sources. Experts estimate that indoor air pollution in many homes is two to ten times worse than outdoor pollution. The interaction of these compounds, as well as the cumulative exposure can have devastating effects. Many of the chemicals in household products cause cancer. Additionally, memory impairment, slowed thinking, headaches, burning sinuses, rashes, joint pain, problems with muscle coordination, irritability, fatigue, and sleep disturbances are reported effects. When these neurotoxins make their way to your brain, it's like a three-alarm fire on memory cells.

"Sick building syndrome" as it has been called, tends to occur when a home or office is sealed up tightly and has poor ventilation. The toxic fumes from building supplies are trapped and constantly being inhaled.

Walls

Walls beneath plaster board (sheet rock) are usually made from either pressed board or plywood. Pressed board, also called particle board, is made from a mixture of wood chips and sawdust that are compressed into a solid mass and glued with a urea formaldehyde resin. Plywood is made from thin sheets of wood that are laminated together with phenol formaldehyde resin. The toxic fumes from both types of formaldehyde harm the central nervous system; they first compromise the mucous membranes of the nasal passages and lungs, and when formaldehyde gets into the blood, neurological function is at risk.

Wall insulation materials may also contain urea formaldehyde. When installing insulation, be sure to ask the manufacturer for the *The Materials Safety Data Sheet* on insulation. Prepared by the Occupational Safety and Health Administration (OSHA), this bulletin lists the chemical off-gassing levels of various insulation products. Select the one with the lowest emissions. There are over 30,000 of these data sheets on different hazardous materials.

When buying a pre-existing home, find out from contractors what kind of building materials were used in its construction. Make every attempt to discover neurotoxic construction materials before you move in.

Formaldehyde

A multipurpose chemical, formaldehyde is found in disinfectants, preservatives, and glues. Urea-formaldehyde resin, the adhesive used in plywood and pressed-board building supplies, emits toxic fumes. The off-gassing of supplies made with formaldehyde is associated with headaches, nausea, concentration problems, memory loss, and general neurotoxic damage.

In addition to building supplies, formaldehyde is also present in magazine and book bindings, pressed-board furniture, plastic items, and carpet glues. It is also used as a disinfectant and general preservative. Carpenters in their twenties and thirties, who are constantly around formaldehyde, have complained of impaired mental ability, forgetfulness, inability to concentrate, and unprovoked irritability. Formaldehyde and other adhesives are suspect. Funeral directors use formaldehyde as an embalming agent. Remember that rubbery looking frog you dissected back in the eighth grade? It was preserved in formaldehyde.

Household Items

A number of common household items can be a source of dangerous neurotoxins. Although seemingly harmless, furniture, carpeting, and even wall coverings can emit toxic fumes, putting your health at risk.

Pressed-Board Furniture

Inexpensive, pressed-board furniture is a health risk because of the toxic adhesives used in its production. As mentioned earlier, pressed wood is made from a compressed mixture of wood chips and sawdust that are held together with a toxic resin. Most pieces of furniture made with pressed board are generally covered with formica or a thin sheet of wood called a laminate. The adhesives used to bind these coverings to the pressed board are generally toxic, adding to the harmful off-gassing of the furniture. If you do purchase chairs, tables, cabinets, dressers, or any other furniture that is made with pressed board, be sure to brush any exposed areas with a clear, nontoxic sealer.

Floor Coverings

The latex backing on many rugs and carpets contains 4-phenylcyclohexene, a neurotoxic substance that can elicit such reactions as respiratory problems, headaches, and skin rashes in some individuals. The off-gassing of this substance also alters message reception in memory cells, to which babies and young children are the most susceptible. Do not allow latex-backed rugs in your home.

When shopping for carpeting, choose only those made of 100 percent wool or nylon. Never buy carpeting that is a synthetic blend, which often contain petrochemicals. And be sure the carpet backing has a coarse, hemp-like backing with no latex or glue between the top fiber and the backing. These top and bottom layers should be stitched together, not glued. Do not be swayed by labeling tactics that *hint* at low neurotoxicity. Carpet companies know consumers are getting wise to toxic emissions.

Some manufacturers add antimicrobial substances to the carpeting to keep insects away. Such chemicals are, of course, neurotoxic pesticides and harmful not only to memory cells, but to immune function in the brain as well. The nose knows. If you smell any foul chemicals in the carpet, move on to another brand. Also, avoid carpeting that has been protected by soil-resistant chemicals. Incorporate the habit of leaving shoes at the door. You will be amazed at how clean your carpets will stay.

The foam padding, commonly used under carpeting, contains a urea formaldehyde that contributes to the neurotoxicity in the home. Always choose felt or cotton fiber padding, instead.

When new carpeting is installed, keep a written record for several months on your family's health. Is anyone getting bad headaches or having dizzy spells with regularity? Is anyone experiencing eye strain, eye puffiness, or post-nasal drip? Has the canary stopped singing? Is the cat suddenly biting your children when it never did before? Have plants died? If these symptoms go away when your family leaves the house, you may have a "sick" carpet.

Avoid using glue to adhere carpeting to the floor. The fumes emitted by carpet glues can have neurotoxic effects that can last for years. Rather tack or staple carpeting to the floor. If floor covering has already been glued down at home or work, try to create your own oasis by placing a Hepa air filter or a fume absorber in the room. And decorate the room with a spider plant or two. Spider plants appear to absorb and actually thrive on formaldehyde fumes.

Instead of carpeting, you might consider opting for old fashioned cloth rag rugs. Flooring made with wood, bricks, or clay tiles are safer alternatives to carpeting or linoleum.

Less toxic glues are now available in some hardware stores. Read glue and adhesive labels. If you must use glue, be sure the product you select does not contain neurotoxins like acetone, benzene, ketones, toluene, or xylene. Whenever possible, minimize the use of neurotoxic adhesives in your home and workplace.

Paints

The solvents and chemicals used in interior wall paint fill the air with noxious fumes. These fumes have been known to cause drowsiness, nausea, headaches, and asthmatic attacks. Some paints contain herbicides to fight the mold and fungi that can grow under paint. Some oil-based paints can take up to three months to dissipate.

The good news is that now, nontoxic paints—free of chemicals like benzene, ketones, toluene, and tricholoroethylene—are readily available. Dulex paint manufacturer, for instance, offers a paint that contains no volatile organic compounds (VOC).

If you believe mold growth may be a problem (in an old bathroom, for instance) try not to give up and use a paint with an herbicide. Instead, scrub the walls well with a nontoxic cleanser such as Murphy's Oil Soap. Remember to rinse it well, then allow the walls to dry before applying the nontoxic paint. This may seem like a lot of work, but it is better than using paint with a strong herbicide that may hang around for years. Making one's home beautiful and comfortable is a worthy consideration, but not at the expense of neurological health.

Electromagnetic Fields

The average man or women probably never gives a second thought to the safety of their bedside electric clock radio, sewing machine, or TV. But such electrical sources emit invisible, weightless forces known as electromagnetic fields (EMFs). And low-level exposure to EMFs has been implicated in a number of serious health conditions including chronic fatigue syndrome, miscarriages, and certain cancers, as well as dementia and severe memory loss.

Natural fields that generate both electric and magnetic radiation are generated by the planets, the sun, the moon, and by every living thing, including our own bodies. Our bodies are regulated and attuned to the Earth's field, and they pulse at about the same rate. However, *artificial* electromagnetic fields—waves radiated from just about everything connected to an electric circuit—pulse at a different rate. The currents in these pulsating waves move back and forth in an alternating pattern. And it is this movement that may be interfering with the body's own electrical current, disturbing cell membranes.

Human studies show a connection between EMFs and brain tumors, as well as other neurological disturbances. Researchers involved in studies at the University of Southern California reported an increased risk of severe memory loss that is characteristic of Alzheimer's disease in people who worked most of their lives on electric sewing machines. A joint study between Canadian and French researchers in 1993, analyzed the health histories of over 223,000 electrical workers. They discovered those who had the most direct contact with electromagnetic fields were twelve times more likely to develop brain tumors than those workers with less EMF exposure. A similar study involving 138,000 utility workers found a direct association between EMFs and brain cancer.

Important research involving lab animals performed by the

Department of Bioengineering at the University of Washington found that low-level microwave radiation decreases the acetylcholine activity that moves memory in the hippocampus of the brain. These same researchers have found that exposure to low-frequency EMFs over a long period of time can cause breaks in the genetic information in cellular DNA, weaken spatial learning ability, and lower intelligence.

The cells making up memory neurons are like other cells in the body. They weaken with time and become more susceptible to physical stress. Until more definitive studies are conducted, why take chances? Develop a healthy respect for the possible neurological effects of transformers and other sources of electromagnetic fields. The National Institute of Environmental Health Sciences and the U.S. Department of Energy offer a number of protective suggestions against EMFs in the home and workplace:

- Distance yourself from EMF sources. Keep a distance of six feet or more from television sets, refrigerators, freezers, and electrical heaters; and at least one foot from hair dryers. Sit two to three feet from the front of computer monitors.

- Don't let children play near outdoor power lines or transformers.

- When an electrical source is not in use, turn it off and unplug it. As long as an electrical source is plugged in, the wires are "hot," and power is flowing through them.

- Place dial-faced electric clocks at least four feet from your bed. Keep digital models at least six feet away.

- Get an EMF shield for your computer monitor as well as your television set. Sold in electronics stores, these shields can help reduce the magnetic emissions.

- Whenever possible, use battery-operated appliances rather than electric ones.

- Do not use remote devices such as cordless and cellular telephones, or those used for garage doors, televisions, VCRs, or toys. They tend to generate strong EMFs.

To measure the EMF level in your home or neighborhood, contact an environmental testing service or consider purchasing a gaussmeter—an easy-to-use device that measures both indoor and outdoor EMFs. For a listing of gaussmeter sales centers, send $1.00 and a self-addressed stamped envelope to *Microwave News*, PO Box 1799, Grand Central Station, New York, NY 10163. This newsletter also details how the home and work environment can be made more user friendly around electrical equipment. You might suggest that your local library subscribes to this excellent resource.

For more information on EMFs from a historical and scientific viewpoint, read *Cross Currents* by Dr. Robert O. Becker, M.D. (New York: St. Martin's Press, 1990). The consumer's guide *Electromagnetic Fields* by B. Levitt (New York: Harcourt Brace & Co., 1995) presents suggestions on how to protect oneself from EMFs in the home and workplace. To obtain a free copy of *Questions and Answers about EMFs* by the National Institute of Environmental Health Sciences, call 1–800–363–2383.

IN SUMMARY

Make no mistake. The neurotoxic sources covered in this chapter are for real. They carry serious neurological risks. Awareness of these and other factors presented in this book can help you make necessary changes in the way you live. Remember, the more neurotoxic dangers you remove from your life, the better your memory and general health will be in years to come.

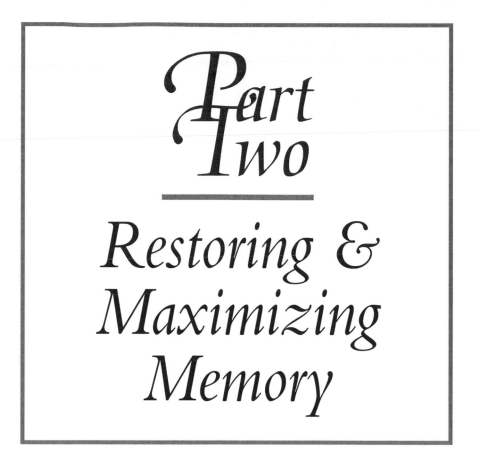

Part Two

Restoring & Maximizing Memory

N ow that you have learned how memory works, as well as the many causes for its failure, it is time to take action. Start with an honest look at the extent of your memory loss, then decide on the best course of action to restore it. The chapters in Part Two will help you achieve this goal.

Part Two begins with Chapter 5, which is designed to help you assess your memory loss. It includes a three-part questionnaire to help you determine if you can deal with your memory problem through certain lifestyle adjustments, such as nutritional supplementation and cellular detoxification, or whether consulting a memory specialist is the most prudent course of action. Chapters 6 and 7 present the many nutrients and pharmaceutical products that have shown success in helping support and restore memory loss. Finally, a variety of detoxification treatments, including chelation and oxygen therapies, detox saunas, and juice fasts, are presented. Part Two concludes with a summarization of the various strategies you can use to help boost your memory.

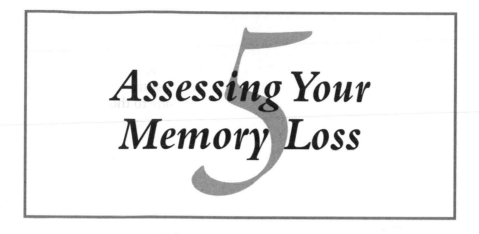

Assessing Your Memory Loss

"Worry is the interest paid on trouble before it falls due."

—W.R. Inge

*T*he ideal memory restoration program is a tailor-made plan designed for your needs alone. What works for a family member or friend may not be the best course of action for you. This chapter offers a simple questionnaire to help you determine the extent of your memory loss.

STAGES OF NATURAL MEMORY LOSS

With the exception of amnesia caused by strokes or severe head injuries, most memory loss takes place over a gradual period of time. When it is faced early enough, you have both the time and opportunity to do something about it. The tests presented in this chapter are designed to help you analyze natural memory loss, not the more severe memory loss associated with Alzheimer's disease and senile dementia.

Of course, such assessments are not perfect and are not meant to build a hysterical case against your memory. Rather, they are presented as indicators of a possible problem; they can help motivate you to take action before a more serious problem develops. Most people will find that they fall well within the boundaries of natural memory loss; however, should you feel that your memory loss lies beyond these categories, by all means, seek professional help.

According to the Global Deterioration Scale, developed by Dr. Barry Reisberg, clinical director of the Aging and Dementia Research Center at the New York University Medical Center, memory decline can be categorized into seven distinct stages, ranging from the normal memory function of stage one to the severe memory loss of stage seven. Early age-associated memory loss begins with stage two—normal age-related forgetfulness—then it progresses to stage three—mild, early memory decline. Stages four through seven are associated with memory loss stemming from Alzheimer's disease or other forms of dementia. Stages two and three are the phases we are concerned with here.

The age-related memory loss experienced during stage two of memory decline is very mild—but very real, nonetheless. A person may, for example, begin to forget the names of people he or she knows well, or misplace familiar items, like house keys or beepers, with increasing regularity. A person in this stage of memory decline may have difficulty remembering a seven-digit phone number the first time he or she hears it. Often this memory loss is so mild it may not manifest itself in work or social situations. Friends, family, and coworkers may not even notice the signs, or they may blame the cognitive slips on stress and fatigue. The person experiencing the loss, however, is likely to at least begin to feel concern.

Mild to moderate memory decline in overall cognitive function characterizes the third stage of early age-related memory loss. Memory deficits are rather clear and well defined. A person in this stage may forget how to get to a seldom-traveled location, or his or her work performance may decline. Other common signs of stage three memory loss include difficulty in mental concentration, a declining ability to perform under stressful working conditions, and mild to moderate anxiety over the weakening memory. Trouble with reading retention is also typical during this stage.

If you experience any of the signs just mentioned, don't assume you are experiencing early Alzheimer's disease. Remember, only a very small percentage of the population is actually diagnosed with this illness. Most people who experience memory problems fall into stage two or stage three categories, and in most cases, these stages are reversible. You must, however, be willing to make some definite changes in your life—nutritional dietary changes and lowered stress levels, for example. If you are experiencing stage three symptoms or more severe signs of memory loss, it is important that you have a complete neurological assessment by a doctor who is trained in memory disorders.

MEMORY QUESTIONNAIRE

The following questionnaire is designed to help you determine the degree and seriousness of your memory problem. These simple questions are based on the memory assessment concepts found in Dr. Reisberg's Global Deterioration Scale (discussed on page 96). Divided into three parts, this survey will help you decide how well your memory functions are serving you. Look at small changes in memory that may be signaling a warning. Whatever you do, don't panic! Just be sure to view this questionnaire as an early warning device for needed lifestyle changes. Simple changes today can avoid serious memory problems in the future.

Whether you have perfect memory, mild forgetfulness, or memory that is in need of help, this test can help indicate subtle issues that need to be addressed. Be sure to score each of the following questions as accurately as possible, using the following scale:

**Never = 0   Seldom = 1   Sometimes = 2
Often = 3   Always = 4**

PART I

1. In order to write down a phone number from an answering machine, I have to replay the message more than once. _____

2. I lose my pen a lot. _____

3. Seconds after meeting someone, I forget his or her name, even if it is someone I should be remembering. _____

4. I can't remember where I went on my last vacation. _____

5. After looking up a telephone number, I need to write it down before I can make the call. _____

6. I go to a room in my home and do not know why I went there. _____

7. The day after an important meeting, I have to refer to my notes to remember the points covered. _____

8. After pressing clothes, I forget to unplug the iron.   _____

9. After dialing a phone number, I forget who I called and why.   _____

10. I am concerned about my inability to remember little things.   _____

                                                  Total Part I _____

PART II

1. I have trouble finding my car in large parking lots.   _____

2. Finding the way back to the hotel on my vacation is difficult.   _____

3. I forget to turn off running faucets after I wash my hands.   _____

4. I forget to finish tasks that I have started.   _____

5. It is difficult for me to retain new information.   _____

6. People tell me they have met and spoken to me, but I can't remember ever meeting them.   _____

7. I forget to feed my child or my pet.   _____

8. After returning from the grocery store, I realize I have forgotten to get the item I had originally gone there for.   _____

9. I forget important topics I have discussed with family members.   _____

10. I am anxious about my memory loss and try to hide it from others.   _____

                                                 Total Part II _____

PART III

1. After experiencing a reaction to food, I am more forgetful than usual.   _____

2. I have trouble remembering "little things" after receiving anesthesia for a diagnostic procedure.   _____

3. I forget the way home after I have been drinking alcohol. _____

4. My memory seems worse at the end of the day. _____

5. I use recreational drugs like marijuana and/or cocaine. _____

6. Professional exterminators treat my house at least once every two years for termites or other insects. _____

7. I crave sweets, starches, and fruit juices. _____

8. I eat meals in fast food outlets, cafeterias, and restaurants. _____

9. When I get a dental filling, it is usually mercury amalgam. _____

10. I take antibiotics or nonsteroidal anti-inflammatory medicine. _____

Total Part III _____

Total Sum _____

Scoring Your Answers

Add up the scores for Parts I, II, and III. Each part will total between 0 and 40. Next, add the scores from all three parts for a total sum. Here, your score will range from 0 to 120. An overall total score of 36 suggests the beginning stages of memory loss. It is wise at this point to begin making some lifestyle changes to help prevent your memory loss from escalating.

Begin with a complete physical examination from a qualified health-care practitioner, preferably one who is well-versed in treating memory problems. Be sure to discuss any drugs or medications you may be taking. Together, discuss certain lifestyle adjustments presented in this book that may be able to reverse your memory loss. For instance, avoid fast-foods, processed foods, and foods containing chemical additives and flavor enhancers. Have your hair analyzed for possible heavy metal contamination, and, depending on the results, take steps to eliminate the metals from your system. Avoid proximity to electrical appliances. Stop eating foods with refined sugar. Do not use products containing aluminum (including cookware and utensils), baking powder, deodorant, or laxatives. Together, develop a nutritious meal plan that includes lots of enzyme-rich raw fruits and vegetables, as well as daily vitamin and mineral supplements. Reduce stress levels in your life.

Men and Women Score Differently on Memory Tests

Memory assessment expert Thomas Crook has examined hundreds of people over the years. He has made the following observations about important cognitive differences between the sexes:

- *Women tend to score higher on learning and memory tests than do men.* This does not mean women are brighter than men, it simply means that these activities hold more meaning for them. Men are likely to focus on attaining a goal, and once the goal is achieved, they move on to another. Generally, they do not spend a lot of time thinking about and remembering an event. Women, on the other hand, love discussing *all* the details of the experiences that fill their days.

- *Men tend to process incoming signals from the outside world with less emotion than do women.* One common exception, however, is in the arena of sports. Here, men know exactly how they feel about Tiger Woods or Pete Rose in strong emotional terms. So never assume that men do not "feel." They simply process and store these signals in different ways than women do.

- *Women tend to remember details of the emotion for years.* Men are inclined to "move on" with their emotions and often cannot tell you how they feel about an event that happened last month unless it involved a life or death issue. This may be why some men forget anniversaries and birthdays. They tend to process such information in a more linear pattern—"here's how I handled it; here's how it turned out."

  A woman and man can experience the same event and perceive it differently. For instance, when Cammy and her husband made their first trip to Paris, she bought a lovely French suit with matching purse, shoes, and, yes, gloves. Cammy still has the shopping bag she used to carry these purchases, while her husband would have dumped it long ago. Cammy does not care that the bag serves no purpose. For her, it contains a meaningful memory.

- *Men have a tendency to focus on the task at hand, and will concentrate on attaining that goal.* Women, on the other hand, tend to juggle multiple tasks at once with little effort.

If a man and woman can partner their particular learning and memory tendencies together, they are likely to conquer anything.

CONCLUSION

Although you may have to face the fact that you have some memory problems, know that you can begin to take steps to recover that lost memory and prevent any future memory loss. Don't allow memory function to deteriorate to the point of no return. If you learn nothing else from this book, know that it is better to start a memory restoration program sooner than later.

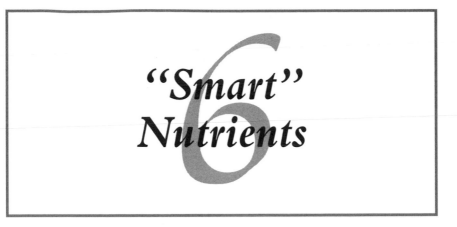

"Smart" Nutrients

"An ounce of prevention is worth a pound of cure."
—Ancient Jewish Teaching

*K*enneth is studying for his entrance exam to get into law school, only he is on edge. Always a straight "A" student as an undergraduate math major, Kenneth is struggling with a calculus review course. At thirty-seven years old, he's having trouble with equations he once found so easy. Concentration is a problem too. A recent physical showed Kenneth to be in good health. His doctor suggested a prescription for anxiety, but Kenneth wants more than a pill to solve his vague cognitive problem.

For Jan, life at the office is a living nightmare. A bookkeeper, Jan still has two years before retirement and doesn't know how she is going to survive them. Her memory is shot. People call her on the phone and rattle off numbers, but Jan can't get them all down before she has to ask for a repeat. Agenda items from important office meetings are a blur in her mind. Jan's forty-something boss is pressing to get her fired. Jan is frantic about her forgetfulness.

Kenneth and Jan, though separated by a generation, are both ideal candidates for memory-enhancing nutrients. Fortunately, such nutrients targeted for cognitive and memory regeneration now exist to support the brain in its functions.

YOUR MEMORY ENGINE

Think of memory as a factory that is made up of hundreds of tiny motors that move thoughts around twenty-four hours a day, every day. In order for these motors to do an effective job, they need specific types of cellular fuels for energy. Low levels of cell energy cause cerebral neurons to falter during memory activity.

As the years pass, memory tissue becomes more vulnerable to aging factors. Pollution, stress, and disease all take a toll on the nerve tissues in your brain. Enzyme defenses enjoyed in youth drop to increasingly lower levels during midlife. Cell membranes that control enzyme flow become less flexible and more rigid. Mineral ions that support memory flow cannot pass through membrane walls as easily as they once did. The setting is right for a dramatic increase in free radical damage. As these oxidizing factors line up for attack, an aging cell with low-energy and low-sugar levels is less able to resist them.

At such a time, it is important to give your neurons a "second chance" at life with substances to help increase cellular energy. We call these cell building blocks and fuels—enzymes, amino acids, essential fats, vitamins, and minerals—"smart" nutrients because they enhance your thought and memory pathways by feeding and repairing the neuronal environment. Though each of these nutrients performs in different ways, their common goal is to preserve and extend memory.

To help keep your body nutritionally sound it is important to eat nutrient-rich, well-balanced meals. Knowing what to eat is as important as knowing what foods to avoid. Supplementing your diet with vitamins and other "smart nutrients" is another way to help keep your body and mind in good working order.

THE IMPORTANCE OF ENZYMES

Although detailed information on memory-enhancing supplements is presented in this chapter, know that eating the right foods is just as important. The vitamins, minerals, and protein chains needed for good memory are held together by enzymes that act as switches for the important chemical reactions of memory.

Protein-based enzymes play a necessary role in virtually all of the biochemical activities that go on in the body. They are essential for digesting food, for stimulating the brain, for providing cellular energy, and for repairing tissues, organs, and cells.

Enzymes fall into two basic categories: metabolic and digestive. Metabolic enzymes play a part in all body processes, including breathing, moving, thinking, and maintaining the immune system. They help neutralize poisons and carcinogens such as tobacco smoke and other environmental pollutants. Digestive enzymes, which are primarily manufactured by the pancreas, are necessary in breaking down the bulk of partially digested food that leaves the stomach. They also aid in the bodily absorption of the food's important nutrients.

While the body manufactures a supply of digestive enzymes, it can also obtain these enzymes from raw foods. Enzyme research has revealed the importance of a diet that is rich in raw foods—specifically fresh fruits, vegetables, and grains. These enzymes are crucial for the bodily absorption of vitamins and minerals.

Enzymes found in raw foods, however, are extremely sensitive to heat. Even relatively low heat (118°F) destroys most of these enzymes. A diet composed exclusively of foods that are cooked, processed, or sugar-laden puts a strain on the pancreas. If the pancreas is constantly overstimulated to produce the enzymes that should come from food, the eventual result will be inhibited function. This can lead to shortened lifespan, illness, and lowered resistance to stress.

Eating raw foods or taking enzyme supplements helps prevent the depletion of the body's own enzymes. This reduces stress on the body. Avocados, papayas, pineapples, bananas, and mangos are all high in enzymes. Sprouts are a rich source, as are cabbage, wheatgrass, Brussels sprouts, broccoli, and most green plants.

Scientists are unable to manufacture enzymes synthetically. Supplemental digestive enzymes are generally made from animal enzymes, such as pancreatin and pepsin, which aid in the digestion of food and the absorption of important nutrients.

TAKING SMART NUTRIENT SUPPLEMENTS

Before taking smart nutrients, first examine your individual cognitive needs. Then, target those conditions with a supplement that is specifically designed to meet that purpose. Generally, these nutrients will either increase energy levels, maintain blood glucose, build immune strength, or prevent the destructive oxidation of neurons by free radicals. As each nutrient performs a different task, it may be necessary to take more than one of these memory-enhancing substances. Sometimes smart-nutrient combinations are more effective than one supplement taken alone.

Before taking any nutritional supplement, it is important to be checked by a qualified health-care practitioner to determine if you have sensitivities to it. If you discover that you are allergic to a supplement needed to enhance your cognitive and memory function, it is important to eliminate that sensitivity. Allergic reactions can be minimized and even eliminated in most cases (see NAET method in Chapter 9). When the body is allergic to a substance, it tries to eliminate that substance quickly. This means that no matter how much of a vitamin, enzyme, or mineral you take, if you are allergic to it, the substance will be excreted before it is absorbed.

If you do not replenish nutritional fuels for the brain, your thinking, learning, and memory ability will start to slow down and eventually disappear. Even worse, if nutritional support is weak, the neurons will be more vulnerable to the overstimulating effects of the excitotoxins that are used in many foods to enhance flavor. With continual overstimulation, these memory cells burn up and die. As large numbers of neurotransmitter pathways are destroyed, the risk for significant memory loss increases.

SMART NUTRIENTS FROM A TO Z

The following smart nutrients are designed to improve current cognitive levels of operation and increase memory longevity. These important elements can help cut the risk of severe memory loss as you age. Together with your health-care practitioner decide which of the following supplements may be helpful to you and your specific needs.

Acetylcarnitine

The amino acid acetylcarnitine (acetyl-L-carnitine) is a special protective agent for memory. Derived from the L-carnitine found in all living cells, acetylcarnitine is a great friend to the nervous system. It moves memory through neurons and across synaptic gaps in a way that is similar to the major neurotransmitter acetylcholine.

Made naturally in the human liver, kidney, and brain, acetylcarnitine improves learning performance and memory retrieval in older people and slows cognitive decline. This special neurotransmitter also helps clean out free radicals, increase neuronal energy levels, and protect the stability of the blood-brain barrier against harmful substances. For instance, acetylcarnitine can "chelate" or draw excess amounts of harmful iron out of memory cells.

Experimental studies have shown that acetylcarnitine can reverse damage to memory cells in the hippocampus—the first stop for information storage and retrieval in the brain. It also reduces age pigment accumulation and promotes the movement of choline in the memory pathways. When information moves smoothly and quickly, memory flows normally.

In one study, Alzheimer's patients who were treated with acetylcarnitine showed less cognitive and memory deterioration than age-matched Alzheimer's patients who were not treated. Another study notes that acetylcarnitine works better in early-onset memory loss in people under sixty-five years old than in those over sixty-five. And patients who were treated with acetylcarnitine after stroke recovered faster and did not lose as much weight as stroke victims not given this supplement.

Certain areas of memory tissue are sensitive to various kinds of neurotransmitters, a necessary feature to give memory function the vast flexibility needed for thought. Such areas are called *receptors* and are crucial for good memory. But as the years go by, neuron receptors weaken and eventually die, causing holes to develop in memory tissue. Acetylcarnitine helps slow down the destruction of memory receptors in the hippocampus. The inflammation caused by the herpes simplex virus seems to strike these areas in the hippocampus, bringing about the danger of short-term memory loss. For this reason, herpes sufferers can benefit from the neuronal protective quality of acetylcarnitine.

Acetylcarnitine is found naturally in certain foods such as red meat and dairy products, but in order to receive an effective amount, supplementation is necessary.

Acetylcarnitine has a wide variety of positive effects on the memory body, including the following:

- Defends memory tissue against free radical damage.

- Crosses the blood-brain barrier with ease.

- Supports the work of acetylcholine.

- Reverses neuron loss in key memory areas of the hippocampus and prefrontal area of the cerebrum.

- Enhances message flow between the two hemispheres of the brain.

- Increases levels of the antioxidants glutathione and coenzyme Q_{10} in memory lobes.

- Offers herpes sufferers some protection against destruction of short-term memory in the hippocampus.

- Protects the neuronal receptors in the hippocampus that MSG and other excitotoxins tend to destroy.

- Safeguards electron transport and restores oxidative damage to the inner membranes of the mitochondria (the energy furnace inside the memory cells), providing more fuel to power memory.

- Encourages the manufacture of proteins inside the mitochondria.

- Reverses damage to the transfer mechanism between DNA and RNA in gene code signaling.

- Increases GABA, an inhibitory neurotransmitter that prevents overstimulation of memory receptors.

Recommended Dosage

People under age fifty who have only slight or no memory loss might start out taking 250 milligrams of acetylcarnitine three times a day. For those suffering from substantial memory decline, 1.5 to 3 grams of acetylcarnitine a day is recommended. For more severe memory loss, the recommended daily dosage is 3 to 4 grams.

Do not take acetylcarnitine in one large dose. For best results, divide it into three doses a day and take it before meals. As acetyl-carnitine is eliminated from the body within ninety minutes, 500 milligrams of choline is also recommended to be taken with each dose to help reduce urinary elimination. If you are also taking phosphatidyl serine (page 129), you can reduce the recommended dosage of each. These two smart nutrients are more powerful in the presence of each other.

Cautionary note: While no serious side effects from acetylcarnitine have been reported, a small number of people have experienced "agitation." If you have this reaction, try taking acetylcarnitine after meals, which may prevent this effect. If this doesn't help, either lower the dose or stop taking the substance.

Alpha-Lipoic Acid

When blood supply is cut off to the brain (even for just a few minutes), such as the result of a stroke or cardiac arrest, large numbers of free radicals attack neurons. Studies show that animals that have been given alpha-lipoic acid have a 60 percent lower death rate following oxygen deprivation.

Alpha-lipoic acid preserves memory tissue by increasing glutathione levels, which protect fat stores in neurons from being damaged. Found mostly in body cells, alpha-lipoic acid supports blood flow to vessel-rich neurons in memory tissue. It also encourages nerve regrowth not only in the brain, but throughout the body. It is a powerful antioxidant that helps neutralize free radicals that cause cellular "rusting." Alpha-lipoic acid also protects memory tissue against heavy metal poisoning, as well as variety of destructive changes in the aging cell.

By acting like a light switch, alpha-lipoic acid turns on a cascade of enzymatic reactions that work to protect against the unhealthy interaction of proteins and sugars known as *glycosylation*. Also known as the "browning" effect, glycosylation occurs in diabetes and other cellular aging processes.

Russian children exposed to low-level radiation after the Chernobyl catastrophe showed high levels of free radicals in their blood. But those who were treated with alpha-lipoic acid soon after exposure showed levels that were markedly lower. Those children who were given vitamin E supplements in addition to the alpha-lipoic acid, displayed levels that were even lower, and, in some cases, normal.

So powerful are the effects of alpha-lipoic acid on memory tissue, older test animals outperformed younger animals twenty-four hours after receiving it.

Alpha-lipoic acid has a number of positive effects on the memory body, including the following:

- Helps cellular energy production in neurons by improving the movement of glucose through membranes even when insulin levels are low or nonexistent.

- Regenerates nerve cells in the brain.

- Neutralizes free radicals and prepares them for excretion from the body.

- Increases blood flow in the memory environment.

- Has strong chelating power, pulling harmful heavy metals from the blood that passes through memory tissue.

- Intensifies the action of other antioxidants—particularly vitamins C and E.

- Shields DNA from free radical damage.

- Increases levels of coenzyme Q_{10} and the intracellular antioxidant glutathione to help protect against the aging of brain cells.

- Protects cells that are exposed to aniline dyes, heavy metals, solvents, and various arsenic compounds.

Recommended Dosage

Take 100 to 200 milligrams of alpha-lipoic acid three times a day. For those who have diabetes or suffer from mercury poisoning, take 300 to 600 milligrams three times a day. For greater antioxidant effect, take alpha-lipoic acid with a daily total of 800 IU vitamin E and 1,000 milligrams vitamin C, spread out over three doses. For maximum alpha-lipoic acid potency, also take a daily dose of 50 milligrams each of thiamine and niacin.

Cautionary note: After thirty years of testing alpha-lipoic acid, there have been no reports of adverse side effects.

Boron

Boron enhances brain function and promotes alertness, especially in the elderly, who commonly begin to show slowed memory response and general cognitive decline. This trace mineral is also needed for the absorption of calcium, which is necessary for efficient vitamin B_{12} absorption.

Boron is found in apples, carrots, grapes, leafy vegetables, peas, beans, peaches, and pears. It is also found in whole grains.

There are a number positive effects that boron has on the memory body, including the following:

- Helps balance electrolytes during the production of electrical currents in memory tissue.

- Makes certain enough calcium is present in key memory areas.

- Decreases memory processing time.

- Promotes the absorption of calcium.

Recommended Dosage

Take 3 milligrams of boron daily.

Cautionary note: Too much boron may have an adverse effect on neurons. Do not take more than 3 milligrams a day.

Calcium

Calcium serves as an important messenger within memory cells. It regulates the ability to respond to new learning and store memory for later retrieval.

Maintaining the correct calcium balance does not seem to be affected so much by age as it is by lifestyle and proper nutrition. A person in his or her nineties can and often does show good calcium function, while a younger person might have low levels. Calcium deficiency can cause high blood pressure, increasing the danger of stroke. Too much calcium caused by increased levels of stress hormones in the memory pathway destroys memory neurons.

One way to maintain proper calcium levels is to cut down on salt intake. A New Zealand study established that a high salt diet can flush up to 30 percent of the dietary intake of calcium from the body. Postmenopausal women, who are at a higher risk for osteoporosis than other women, should restrict their salt consumption. They should also avoid foods with flavor enhancers—especially monosodium glutamate (MSG). Alcohol consumption also neutralizes calcium. Be aware that for proper calcium absorption, the trace minerals boron (see page 110) and magnesium (page 122) are necessary in proper ratios.

Calcium is found in milk and other dairy foods, salmon (with bones), sardines, seafood, broccoli, skim milk and other nonfat dairy products, dried figs, soybeans, sesame seeds, tofu, and most beans. Green leafy vegetables like Swiss chard, kale, collard greens, mustard greens, turnip greens, and dandelion greens are also rich sources. Kelp is by far the best source of calcium with nearly 1,100 milligrams per $3\frac{1}{2}$-cup serving (the same amount of milk has 118 milligrams).

Calcium has a number of positive effects on the body that affect memory, including the following:

- Helps control fluid retention and enables the kidneys to release sodium and water, thus reducing the chances of high blood pressure and stroke.

- May control the release of the parathyroid hormone that raises blood pressure.

- Releases neurotransmitters in the memory pathway.

Recommended Dosage

Calcium citrate is the recommended calcium form. Other forms of calcium have been associated with the development of kidney stones. Both men and women alike should take 1,100 milligrams of calcium citrate daily after age forty, and 1,500 milligrams after age fifty. For proper uptake, take calcium in a 2:1 or even a 1:1 ratio with magnesium. For increased calcium uptake, take 3 milligrams of boron with the recommended calcium citrate. Powdered calcium and magnesium combinations are also available. Look for brands that contain lemon or some other acidic base. Use filtered water to mix the powdered form.

Cautionary note: Calcium blocks the medicinal action of the antibiotic tetracycline and may interfere with the effects of verapamil (Calan, Isoptin, Verelan), sometimes prescribed for heart problems and high blood pressure. Calcium supplements should not be taken by those with a history of kidney stones or kidney disease. The FDA warns that calcium derived from bone meal, dolomite, oyster shell, and unrefined calcium carbonate contains high levels of lead. Calcium citrate is the recommended supplemental form. Do not take more than 2,000 milligrams a day.

Choline

Acetylcholine, the brain's main neurotransmitter for memory, comes from choline, which is stored as phosphatidyl choline in neuron bodies and glia cells. One of the B-complex vitamins, choline also encourages the development of new contacts on neuron branches when old contacts are lost. Since new experiences bring new learning, the brain wants to extend its ability to save this information as memory. Choline helps facilitate this new growth and, therefore, the capacity for learning. By such activity, memory is "plastic" and capable of expanding.

Choline encourages the emulsification (even distribution) of fat in the blood, which is a water-based fluid. It also helps prevent cholesterol from sticking to the arterial walls that feed memory tissue. With full blood flow, the chance of oxygen starvation by stroke is lessened in neurons. Nothing kills memory like the absence of oxygen.

Studies at Columbia University discovered that choline brings about long-lasting, positive memory changes in developing neurons of rodents still in the womb. After birth, these choline-fed youngsters had better memory and slower rates of memory decline as they aged than did the offspring of females rats that were not fed choline.

Choline supplementation is an important preventive treatment for memory loss, but supplementation should be started before cholesterol buildup becomes a problem. Some studies have suggested that when a nerve pathway lacks choline, its cell bodies will start digesting their own membranes in a frantic attempt to get more available acetylcholine. This may help to explain the disappearance of massive amounts of memory tissue in the temporal lobes of Alzheimer's patients, who also show very low levels of acetylcholine.

Choline is found in egg yolks, leafy green vegetables, liver, soybeans, yeast, and wheat germ. The best supplemental source of choline is phosphatidyl choline that is derived from soy lecithin. Supplemental free-form choline is not recommended as it must be taken in large quantities, and commonly causes a fishy odor in the breath and perspiration.

Choline has a number of positive effects on the memory body, including the following:

- Changes into acetylcholine, the major neurotransmitter for memory.

- Is absorbed easily through the blood-brain barrier.

- Helps provide energy for "cell signaling," a process that helps tissue duplicate itself and grow.

- Protects and nourishes other chemicals that support memory.

- Encourages a state of calmness.

- Helps control harmful levels of homocysteine, which attack blood vessels.

Recommended Dosage

Take 500 to 1,000 milligrams of choline daily if under age sixty-five. Those over sixty-five should take 1 to 5 grams per day along with 50 milligrams of inositol in a good B-100 vitamin to help with absorption. However, it may be more effective to get choline from lecithin than from choline supplements. For a long-lasting supply of choline for acetylcholine production, take two to three table-spoons of lecithin granules daily. Lecithin also contains small amounts of phosphatidyl serine, another "smart nutrient" for memory.

Be sure to add folic acid, vitamin B_{12}, and methionine supplements with choline for the best results. Most B-complex vitamins contain around 50 milligrams of choline and inositol, but more is required for memory improvement.

Cautionary note: High levels of choline can lower stores of vitamin B_6, so always take B_6 with choline supplements. If not using lecithin as a choline source, look for a choline supplement that also contains inositol. Those in the depressive stage of manic-depressive syndrome should not take choline supplements.

Coenzyme Q_{10}

Coenzyme Q_{10} (CoQ_{10}) plays a critical role in the production of energy in every cell of the body. It aids circulation, stimulates the immune system, and has vital anti-aging effects. In the brain, this coenzyme is extremely important in helping maintain cell energy production for the protection of memory cells. Shortages of CoQ_{10} are linked to primary cardiovascular and cerebrovascular diseases like high blood pressure, angina, and congestive heart failure. Made in the body by phenylalanine and tyrosine, severe shortages of CoQ_{10} result in chronic feelings of fatigue, laziness, and listlessness.

Harvard Medical School studies have established the extensive ability of CoQ_{10} to fight lone oxygen radicals that attack healthy body cells. By increasing CoQ_{10} levels, free radical damage is reduced and blood vessels are less fragile. Studies show that near-ly 40 percent of those with high blood pressure have CoQ_{10} short-ages in cardiovascular tissue. This "smart" nutrient also strength-ens cerebrovascular arterial walls, keeping them from narrowing and closing off the blood supply.

Found largely in salmon, mackerel, and sardines, coenzyme Q_{10} is also contained in beef, peanuts, and spinach. To get maxi-mum benefits, however, CoQ_{10} is best taken in supplement form.

A number of positive effects of coenzyme Q_{10} on the memory body include the following:

- Helps the cell's mitochondria—its energy furnace—produce energy.
- Can lower blood pressure if taken on a regular basis.
- Encourages blood flow in memory tissue.

Recommended Dosage

Take 100 milligrams of coenzyme Q_{10} daily.

Cautionary note: No serious side effects from coenzyme Q_{10} have been reported. Be aware that certain drugs that limit blood cholesterol levels, such as lovastatin, tend to block the formation of coenzyme Q_{10}. Beta-blockers also reduce the enzymes involved in CoQ_{10} processes. When taking such medicines, supplemental coenzyme Q_{10} is especially important.

DMAE (2-dimethylamine ethanol)

When taken with phosphatidyl choline, DMAE helps neuronal tissue produce acetylcholine. This smart nutrient must have both phosphatidyl choline and vitamin B_5 present to produce acetylcholine. DMAE activates the central nervous system as shown by feelings of improved well being. Some scientists believe DMAE's memory-enhancing effects are similar to those produced by the pharmaceutical drug Tacrine. The best way to get DMAE is in supplemental form.

DMAE has a number of positive effects on the memory body, including the following:

- Increases short-term memory.
- Supports concentration powers.
- Enhances ability to learn.
- Improves a sense of well being.

Recommended Dosage

Take 50 to 100 milligrams of DMAE daily. It may take three to four weeks before any memory improvement is noticed.

Cautionary note: If a sense of anxiousness develops after taking DMAE,

Supplemental Estrogen and Memory

Recently, supplemental prescription estrogen has been used by some women to relieve the uncomfortable symptoms of menopause, including hot flashes, vaginal dryness, and mood swings. Some studies have also suggested that estrogen may enhance memory and prevent damage to brain cells. However, estrogen replacement therapy may have a serious dark side that includes a possible link to several forms of cancer.

A 1995 Harvard study, involving 119,000 women over a sixteen-year period, showed a 70 percent greater risk of breast cancer in those women taking supplemental estrogen. Even those women who used this therapy with progestin—the altered form of natural progesterone, which is believed to lower the dangerous side effects of estrogen—still had a 50 percent greater risk of breast cancer than those women who took no supplemental estrogen at all. This estrogen-breast cancer link was reinforced by a report in "The New England Journal of Medicine," while another alarming report implicated long-term estrogen use with an increased risk of ovarian cancer and lupus.

Results like these require serious thought before using estrogen replacement therapy to restore memory or to alleviate uncomfortable menopausal symptoms.

either reduce the intake or stop taking the supplement altogether. As DMAE tends to stimulate nerves, it is best taken early in the day; taken at night, it may cause sleeplessness. This smart nutrient should not be used by anyone with bipolar depression or epilepsy, as it can increase the symptoms of each of these cognitive disorders.

Folic Acid

Considered food for the brain, folic acid is important in neurotransmitter production and in the formation of red blood cells. Sufficient amounts of folic acid along with vitamins B_{12} and B_6 help reduce harmful levels of homocysteine, which can damage the inner walls of blood vessels throughout the circulatory system, including those found in memory tissue. Folic acid is also very important during pregnancy as it helps regulate embryonic and fetal nerve cell formation, which is vital for normal development.

Folic acid is found in whole grains, including barley and brown rice, corn, green leafy vegetables, lentils, oranges, root vegetables, split peas, salmon, tuna, wheat germ, and meats, including beef, chicken, lamb, and pork.

A number of positive effects of folic acid on the memory body include the following:

- Aids in the manufacture of red blood cells, which carry oxygen to memory tissue.

- Regulates fetal development of nerve cells.

- Influences healthy cell division.

- Increases neuron levels of the neurotransmitters serotonin and dopamine.

- Influences many enzymatic and chemical reactions in memory tissue.

- Necessary for stomach acid production, which helps deliver important nutrients to memory tissue.

Recommended Dosage

To protect blood vessels in the brain, take 400 micrograms of folic acid daily. For treating depression, take 10 milligrams divided into several doses throughout the day. To prevent a hidden vitamin B_{12} deficiency, take folic acid with 400 to 1,000 micrograms of vitamin B_{12} daily.

Cautionary note: High doses of folic acid (5 to 10 milligrams) may cause gas, poor appetite, and stomach upset. Those with epilepsy should avoid this supplement in high doses, as it may result in increased seizures. Do not take oral pancreatic enzymes, which tend to reduce folic acid absorption, at the same time as a folic acid supplement. Rather take these two supplements from four to six hours apart. Alcohol, estrogen, chemotherapy, barbiturates, and anticonvulsant drugs also hamper folic acid activity.

Ginkgo Biloba

Ginkgo biloba—an antioxidant herb—comes from the *Ginkgo biloba* tree genus, which has been on earth for 230 million years. Originating in China, this tree now grows in temperate climates through out the world. Ginkgo biloba is excellent in supporting neuronal activity. Hundreds of studies worldwide note that ginkgo helps cognition and memory by protecting and improving blood flow and, therefore, oxygen to the brain. It has the ability to squeeze through even the narrowest of blood vessels.

Among Alzheimer's patients, the effect of ginkgo biloba has been assessed by electroencephalograms (EEGs) and mental function exams. Significant improvement in motor performance and the ability to concentrate and think have been found among some people with such memory loss. In addition, Harvard University studies indicate that lab-produced ginkgolide B, may be promising in the field of organ transplants.

Ginkgo biloba has a number of positive effects on the memory body, including the following:

- Dilates blood vessels in the brain, allowing more oxygenated blood flow to the neurons.

- Protects cerebral tissue when oxygen levels are low.

- Improves short-term memory quickly, when large amounts are taken at one time.

- Keeps blood from clotting.

- May delay the degeneration of memory mass.

Recommended Dosage

Take 40 milligrams of ginkgo biloba three times a day. Look for a product that is guaranteed to be at least 24 percent potent. The standardized extract is more cost-effective and has a higher concentration of neuron-protecting substances than alcohol and alcohol-free tinctures.

Cautionary note: Ginkgo biloba has been used safely in China for over 5,000 years. To date, there have been no known adverse side effects.

Ginseng

Used throughout the Far East as a general tonic to promote energy, ginseng has also been used to enhance athletic performance, to increase longevity, and to normalize the entire system. A general anti-aging substance, ginseng is able to turn off the production of excess cortisol—the stress hormone that burns through memory tissue. Of the many ginseng varieties, American and Siberian are the types generally recommended for restoring balance to an overworked system.

Ginseng has a number of positive effects on the memory body, including the following:

- Increases the production of adrenaline to counteract the presence of cortisol—the damaging stress hormone.

- Helps adrenal function to return to normal after a stressful incident.

- Improves overall stress response in the brain.

Recommended Dosage

For mild memory loss, take 750 milligrams of ginseng daily. For moderate to severe loss, take up to 1,500 milligrams.

Cautionary note: Although ginseng is considered safe, when taken for an extended period of time, it may produce mild side effects, such as insomnia, nausea, excitability, and increased blood pressure, in some individuals.

Glycosaminoglycans

Strokes are caused by the same hardening of the arteries that destroys heart and cardiovascular tissue. It is, therefore, important to maintain strong arteries in memory tissue. Enter glycosaminoglycans (GAGs), which are derived from the amino acid sugar glycosamine. Glycosaminoglycans exist in healthy blood vessels as special sugars known as mucopolysaccharides.

Unlike other forms of body sugar, which are used for energy, GAGs are actually incorporated into the structure of body tissue. Oral forms of GAGs are absorbed with ease into the bloodstream where they are believed to keep arteries strong and healthy.

Neurological symptoms like ringing in the ears, cold hands or feet, depression, headaches, vertigo, and short-term memory loss reflect a lessening of oxygen and blood supply to brain neurons. Research shows GAGs lessen the chance of oxygen shortages by preventing arterial breakdown. Experimental studies have shown them to be more effective than flavonoid extracts, rutosides, and bilberry in protecting vascular structure.

A number of positive effects of glycosaminoglycans on the memory body include the following:

- Protect the inner walls of arteries and veins.

- Increase HDLs (the good cholesterol) levels.

- Aid in the treatment of arterial and vein diseases.

- Help prevent blood clots.

Recommended Dosage

Take 100 milligrams of glycosaminoglycans daily.

Cautionary note: To date, there have been no known adverse side effects from glycosaminoglycans.

Gotu Kola

From the *Centella asiatica* plant, gotu kola is mentioned in ancient Chinese literature. This herb eventually found its way to India, where it became part of Ayurvedic medicine. Indian folk doctors have used gotu kola to treat depression that is caused by physical disorders linked to poor arterial blood flow.

Gotu kola has a number of positive effects on the memory body, including the following:

- Improves vessel wall strength and integrity.

- Increases blood flow to memory neurons.

- Reduces inflammation and swelling of body tissues and cells; promotes healing.

- Soothes nerves.

Recommended Dosage

Take 70 milligrams of gotu kola twice a day.

Cautionary note: Those who should not take gotu kola include pregnant women and anyone with an overactive thyroid.

Green Tea Flavonoids

Many health-giving plant substances fall under the category of flavonoids. One particular group of flavonoids known as polyphenols are found in the fresh tea leaves of the *Camellia sinensis* plant. Both green and black teas come from this plant. Heavy oxidation processing of the *Camellia* leaf, typically used to make black tea, weakens most of the healing power of the polyphenols. But when the leaf is steamed for a few moments, the potent medicinal quality of the fresh plant is saved. Much study has been focused on the cancer-preventing nature of green tea, particularly cancers of the digestive tract, lungs, and breast. Some believe the heavy green tea consumption in Japan accounts for the country's low cancer rates.

The *Camillia sinensis* plant also offers protective effects for memory. The flavonoids found in its green tea leaves help reduce blood clotting and, therefore, decrease the chances of a stroke. They also boost the fight against free radical damage within thirty minutes of consumption. Studies have shown that men who included large amounts of flavonoids in their diet (nearly two-thirds of which came from drinking tea) had more than a 70 percent reduced risk of having a stroke than those men who consumed low flavonoid concentrations. These health-supporting flavonoids are found mostly in green tea leaves and some black tea varieties as well.

The positive effects of green tea flavonoids on the memory body include the following:

• Reduce blood stickiness and clotting factors.

• Lower risk of stroke.

• Support the neuroimmune system.

• Reduce free radical damage.

Recommended Dosages

Several cups of green tea daily are recommended.

Cautionary note: There are no known dangers or harmful side effects from drinking green tea. Those who are sensitive to caffeine, however, may choose to avoid it.

Lecithin

Lecithin is an essential fatty substance that is important to every living cell in the human body. The protective sheaths that surround the brain are composed of lecithin, and the muscles and nerve cells contain lecithin as well. Lecithin enables fats, such as cholesterol and other lipids, to be removed from the body, thus, preventing fatty buildup in vital organs and arteries. In addition to helping prevent arteriosclerosis and cardiovascular disease, lecithin improves brain function.

Supplemental lecithin contains significant amounts of phosphatidyl choline, which stimulates the production of acetylcholine, one of the brain's key neurotransmitters. Lecithin also helps nourish cell membranes, and it provides some protection against harmful free radicals. Lecithin is contained in small amounts in some foods, like soybeans, brewer's yeast, eggs, grains, legumes, red meat, and fish. However, supplemental lecithin granules are more highly concentrated than food sources. Lecithin supplements are highly recommended for those on nonfat or lowfat diets.

The positive effects of supplemental lecithin on the memory body include the following:

- Important in the production of the important neurotransmitter acetylcholine.

- Helps prevent buildup of fats in arteries and vital organs.

- Reduces free radical damage.

Recommended Dosage

Lecithin is a wise addition to anyone's diet. Take 2 tablespoons of lecithin granules daily with food. You can sprinkle them on cereals or soups, or mix them in water or juice. For those with moderate to severe memory loss, take 2 tablespoons of lecithin granules twice daily.

Cautionary note: Although lecithin is considered nontoxic by the FDA, there have been some reports of mild stomach upset in those taking more than 4,000 milligrams a day.

Magnesium

An important mineral for the health of the central nervous system, magnesium is a crucial element in over 300 body reactions. It is a vital catalyst in helping enzymes produce energy and protein for memory neurons, and it also assists in the uptake of calcium and potassium. Magnesium helps maintain proper blood pressure levels by blocking the buildup of calcium inside vessel walls. Studies have shown that magnesium deficiencies increase the risk of free radical damage in certain memory cells. In the Alzheimer's patient, magnesium levels are typically very low.

European studies have demonstrated that a magnesium deficiency increases the chance of death from a heart attack by 50 percent. Studies in Guam established that when aluminum levels are high, magnesium and calcium levels are low. Aluminum is found in cosmetics, laxatives, weight-loss preparations, baking powder, and some food additives, as well as in many cooking utensils.

Magnesium is present in most foods, especially dairy products, fish, meat, and seafood. Apples, avocados, bananas, blackstrap molasses, brewer's yeast, brown rice, garlic, green leafy vegetables, lemons, nuts, sesame seeds, wheat, and whole grains are other excellent sources.

Some of the positive effects of magnesium on the memory body include the following:

- Acts as a catalyst in the energy production in memory neurons.

- Fights free radical damage as a strong antioxidant.

- Minimizes neuronal damage due to insufficient blood.

Recommended Dosage

Take 250 to 350 milligrams of magnesium every day. If pregnant, your doctor may recommend that you take more. For optimum results, take magnesium glycinate, and be sure you take twice as much calcium with it. Some magnesium types, such as magnesium oxide and magnesium sulfate, are not recommended because they are more difficult to absorb into the bloodstream.

Cautionary note: Do not take magnesium after meals as it weakens normal stomach acids. Be aware that the consumption of large quantities of fats, cod liver oil, calcium, vitamin D, and protein decrease magnesium absorption. Fat-soluble vitamins also hinder the absorption of this mineral, as do foods high in oxalic acid, such as almonds, cocoa, rhubarb, and spinach.

Manganese

Manganese helps maintain effective neurotransmitter activity in the brain, boosting good memory. It also improves muscle reflex action, reduces irritability, boosts the immune system, and maintains proper blood sugar regulation. In addition, this important mineral prepares the enzyme activators needed to use vitamin B_1 (thiamine), C, E, and biotin. It is also believed to help those with intestinal problems break down foods. Those who consume large quantities of dairy products as well as meats require increased levels of manganese. High doses of phosphorus and calcium will often stop or slow down the assimilation of manganese.

Rich sources of manganese include avocados, nuts, seeds, and whole grains. It is also found in blueberries, egg yolks, legumes, pineapples, and green leafy vegetables.

Some of the positive effects of manganese on the memory body include the following:

• Crucial for neurotransmitter control.

• Very important for the conversion of glucose into energy within neurons.

• Relieves "lightheadedness" in some people.

Recommended Dosage

Take 1 to 8 milligrams of manganese daily.

Cautionary note: If you experience weakness or find that you have any trouble with muscular movement, cut back on the amount of manganese you are taking. Too much manganese over prolonged periods can limit the amount of iron your body will absorb. In the case of manganese, less may be "better" than more. Also, be aware that large amounts of phosphorus, calcium, bran fiber, and beans can neutralize manganese.

N-Acetyl-L-Cysteine

Although the memory aid N-acetyl-L-cysteine (NAC) comes from the amino acid L-cysteine, it is not an excitotoxin and should not be confused with the flavor enhancer cysteine. NAC increases levels of glutathione, a tripeptide that is important in detoxifying fat-stored toxins such as those from pesticides, solvents, and formaldehyde.

Such fat-stored toxins speed up aging through free radical damage. As long as glutathione levels are high, the cellular damage is kept at a minimum. But as people age, their brains tend to produce less glutathione, making it more and more difficult for memory cells to be protected from free radical damage. The glutathione made from N-acetyl-L-cysteine acts like water on "free-radical fire," while providing increased antioxidant protection for memory tissue.

N-acetyl-L-cysteine is best taken in supplement form. For increased antioxidant power, take NAC with vitamin C.

Many positive effects from N-acetyl-L-cysteine on the memory body include the following:

- Passes with ease into a memory cell where it changes into glutathione, a powerful antioxidant enzyme.

- Breaks up harmful disulfide bonds, making free radical production less destructive.

- Revitalizes the power of vitamin C to scoop up free radicals and sweep them out of the body.

- Decreases the oxidant burden of the oxygen/carbon dioxide exchange mechanism in the lungs, improving the quality of oxygen to memory tissue.

- Helps remove mercury and other toxic metals from body tissue.

Recommended Dosage

Take 500 milligrams of N-acetyl-L-cysteine two times a day with meals.

Cautionary note: No adverse affects of NAC have been reported, even when taken in high doses.

Omega-3 Essential Fatty Acids

Dietary essential fatty acids (EFAs) are crucial for learning and memory because they produce substances that help to limit inflammation in memory cells. Found in large amounts in cerebral tissue, essential fatty acids help message transmission between neurons by keeping the myelin sheath that surrounds nerve cells healthy. Without EFAs, nerve membranes tend to get brittle and inflexible. Essential fatty acids come in various types—the omega 3, 6, 9, and 12 chains.

These essential fats, especially the omega-3 chains, are very important in message transport. They improve the neuron's ability to select which substances may pass in and out of its cell wall. EFAs also help lower cholesterol and maintain normal blood pressure, reducing the risk of stroke. Alpha linoleic acid, which is part of the omega-3 fatty acid chain, has the unique ability to neutralize both water-soluble and fat-soluble neurotoxins in memory tissue.

Essential fatty acids are found in flaxseed oil, black currant oil, grape seed oil, and evening primrose oil. Fish are another source of EFAs. Plant sources of omega-3 fatty acids are generally recommended over those from fish, as they are less likely to contain toxins. However, if you choose a fish oil supplement, it is important that the oil comes from fish, such as cod, that have been caught in deep, cold waters. Certain ocean and fresh water fish, such as swordfish and shark, contain high levels of mercury and other toxic heavy metals. Check the supplement label for a third-party guarantee of the source of the oil.

The highest quality oils from plant sources are expeller pressed from organically grown plants. When choosing oils from plant sources, be sure the product label has a third-party guarantee verifying product quality.

Essential fatty acids have a number of positive effects on the memory body, including the following:

- Appear to heal and protect the flexibility of the membranes that surround neurons, including the blood-brain barrier.

- Help protect fat tissue in the brain from free radical damage.

- Clear certain heavy metals such as cadmium out of the body.

- Help remove mercury from the body by improving bile excretion.

- Reduce stroke potential by limiting hardening of blood vessels that support memory cells in the brain.

- Recycle the powerful free radical fighting antioxidants glutathione and ascorbic acid.

- Improve the connections between neurons in the flow of memory.

- Lower blood cell stickiness, reducing clotting tendencies.

- Regulate blood pressure.

- Help fight inflammation in nerve cells without the harmful gastrointestinal side effects of anti-inflammatory medicine.

- Block the negative effects of the calcium that remains in neuron bodies too long during periods of cortisol secretion and high stress.

Recommended Dosage

Take 1 to 2 tablespoons of a reliable source of omega-3 essential fatty acids for every 100 pounds you weigh. As EFAs are best absorbed when they are taken with vitamins C, E, niacin, and B_6 as well as selenium, magnesium, and zinc, a high-quality multivitamin and mineral supplement is recommended.

Cautionary note: For EFAs to work efficiently, consume no more than 3-ounces of red meat and 3 eggs per week, and reduce intake of dairy products. Diabetics should consult a licensed nutritionist before taking EFA supplementation. Never cook with omega 3 oils.

Phenylalanine

Phenylalanine is an essential amino acid. In the body, phenylalanine is converted into tyrosine, another amino acid that is used to synthesize the neurotransmitters dopamine and norepinephrine. These neurotransmitters promote alertness and vitality, and they are helpful in escorting information across the synaptic gaps between neurons.

Those with Parkinson's disease need increased amounts of dopamine to alleviate the trembling that is characteristic of this disease. For them, phenylalanine is a wise supplement choice. Those who eat a lot of processed foods receive constant, cumulative doses of flavor enhancers, which overexcite memory receptors. Over time, these additives may cause considerable damage to key memory cells in the substantia nigra, resulting in loss of important stabilizing cells for muscle coordination. When cell loss in this area reaches around 70 percent, tremors result.

Phenylalanine supplementation makes good sense, but its presence in your diet does not guarantee that your memory will be protected from dangerous exposure to flavor enhancers and other excitotoxins. The wisest course of action is to eliminate processed foods from your diet.

Phenylalanine is found in pumpkin seeds, sesame seeds, dry skim milk, and lima beans. It is also found in soy products.

Some positive effects of phenylalanine on the memory body include the following:

- Improves memory.

- Increases mental alertness.

- Helps alleviate depression by blocking endorphin-destroying enzymes.

- Is believed to support the substantia nigra from excitotoxin assault.

Recommended Dosage

Take 250 to 500 milligrams of phenylalanine three times daily between meals. Do not take with milk or other proteins. Balance with a reliable brand of free-form amino acids that does not contain L-cysteine, glutamic acid, or aspartic acid.

Cautionary note: Supplemental phenylalanine should not be taken by those who are pregnant, or by those who have high blood pressure, cardio-vascular problems, skin cancer, or phenylketonuria—a genetic inability to convert phenylalanine to tyrosine. Stop taking phenylalanine for four to five consecutive days each month to give memory tissue a rest.

Phosphatidyl Choline

Phosphatidyl choline is important in the production of acetyl-choline—a key neurotransmitter in the brain. It is also helpful in limiting levels of homocysteine, an amino acid that has been implicated in cardiovascular disease. While large amounts of this substance are found in lecithin, supplemental phosphatidyl choline brings better results to early-stage, short-term memory loss.

A number of positive effects of phosphatidyl choline on the memory body include the following:

- Improves acetylcholine production, which helps support message flow in memory cells.

- Protects the outside cell walls of neurons.

- Limits harmful levels of the amino acid homocysteine.

- Supports enzymes that coordinate neurotransmitter production and release.

- Improves the energy supply mechanisms in memory cells.

- Helps memory neurons and glia cells metabolize blood sugar.

- Improves the speed of messages traveling through neurons.

- Maintains the "fluidity" of cell membranes.

Recommended Dosage

Take one 900 milligram soft-gel capsule of phosphatidyl choline, three times daily.

Cautionary note: In some cases, phosphatidyl choline may cause mild stomach upset. If this occurs, reduce the dosage.

Phosphatidyl Serine

A type of lipid or fat found in abundance in all body cells, phosphatidyl serine occurs in the highest amounts in neuronal membranes, where it is able to pass through cell membranes with ease. Because of this trait, phosphatidyl serine helps food enter memory cells; it also helps with the removal of metabolic waste. This action takes place because phosphatidyl serine tends to keep cell membranes permeable for gas and liquid transport on both sides of the cell wall. It also penetrates deep in neuronal tissue to enter each cell's special energy center, where it helps the mitochondria use fuel for memory activity.

One study showed that phosphatidyl serine lowers stress hormone levels significantly. Other research has demonstrated that it encourages a sense of calm by raising the levels of alpha brain waves and increasing the production of acetylcholine. Memory-deficient patients in their mid-sixties who took phosphatidyl serine scored better on cognitive tests than patients who took ginkgo biloba.

The PET scan of one woman with severe cognitive loss showed many areas of reduced electrical activity in her brain. After taking phosphatidyl serine for three weeks, another PET scan was taken and revealed a noticeable increase in cognitive activity. Before this supplementation, many areas of the woman's neuronal tissue had been metabolizing almost twice the amount of sugar than they did after supplementation. While ginkgo biloba helps blood flow in memory tissue, it has not been shown to penetrate and revitalize neuron cells in the manner of phosphatidyl serine.

Phosphatidyl serine is found in lecithin, but needs to be extracted to provide the amounts needed for therapeutic memory restoration. It is best taken in capsule form.

The many positive effects of phosphatidyl serine on the memory body include the following:

• Brings a significant, almost dramatic turnaround in thought and memory function in those experiencing age-based memory impairment.

• Allows memory neurons to conduct nerve impulses more effectively.

• Encourages the release of proper levels of chemical message carriers in memory neurons.

• Helps alleviate depressive symptoms in many patients diagnosed with clinical depression.

• Supports the delivery of acetylcholine to memory neurons.

• Improves the speed and quality of memory transmission in those who have never experienced memory loss.

• Improves the overall ability to think, focus, concentrate, and recall information.

Recommended Dosage

Take 100 to 300 milligrams of phosphatidyl serine daily, depending on the severity of memory loss.

Cautionary note: There are no reported toxicities or negative side effects from phosphatidyl serine.

Selenium

Since two-thirds of cerebral memory and support tissue is made up of fat, it is important to keep this fat from oxidizing in the brain neurons. Considered one of the most important antioxidants for good memory, the trace mineral selenium is a powerful natural quencher of single oxygen radicals that lead to fat-based free radical damage. It also helps the body produce another memory stabilizer—thyroid hormone.

Unfortunately, after age sixty, selenium levels start to decline, limiting its protective effect on fat in and around memory tissue. The typical seventy-year-old will have only 80 percent of the selenium levels characteristic of normal memory in younger people. Men seem to need more selenium than women.

Selenium is found in brewer's yeast, broccoli, brown rice, chicken, dairy products, liver, onions, seafood, tomatoes, wheat germ, and whole grains.

The many positive effects of selenium on the memory body include the following:

- Reduces blood clotting.

- Helps prevent vascular damage, limiting the possibility of a stroke.

- Works with vitamin E to inhibit free radical damage to cell membranes.

- Helps improve arterial circulation in the brain.

- Supports the endocrine and immune centers located in the cerebrum.

Recommended Dosage

Take 50 to 80 micrograms of selenium daily. Give children 1.5 micrograms per pound of weight. Do not exceed 1,000 micrograms in a day.

Cautionary note: As with any trace mineral, be careful not to take too much. Overdoses of selenium can lead to a persistent garlic taste in the mouth, vomiting, depression, and mood swings. High doses of vitamin C can neutralize the potency of selenium.

Vitamin B_1 (Thiamine)

Important for memory, vitamin B_1 is a key substance in a number of metabolic activities. Because one-fourth of the body's metabolic effort takes place in the brain, vitamin B_1 is especially important for good memory. It gives neurons the important building blocks they need for energy production. Epileptic patients taking the drug Dilantin (phenytoin) have noted improved mental function with vitamin B_1 supplementation.

The richest sources of vitamin B_1 include brewer's yeast, brown rice, egg yolks, fish, legumes, liver, nuts, peas, pork, potatoes, poultry, rice bran, wheat germ, and whole grains.

Vitamin B_1 has a number of positive effects on the memory body, including the following:

- Helps increase neuronal energy levels.

- Acts as a strong antioxidant in neuronal tissue.

- Improves blood flow in memory tissue.

- Supports acetylcholine in memory tissue.

- Helps mental processes in Alzheimer's patients.

Recommended Dosage

Take 50 milligrams of vitamin-B complex two times a day—once in the morning and again in the evening. Some people tolerate these vitamins better with food.

Cautionary note: Too much vitamin B_1 can deplete a number of other B vitamins, including B_6. Also, excessive amounts of vitamin B_1 can disrupt insulin and thyroid production. Anyone with a thiamine deficiency who is taking alpha-lipoic acid should supplement with vitamin B_1. Pregnant women should not take vitamin B_1.

Vitamin B_3 (Niacin, niacinamide, nicotinic acid)

This multi-talented B vitamin assists in the production of neurotransmitters and is known to reduce cholesterol levels. Niacin improves circulation in the brain, is effective in treating various mental illnesses, and helps overall neuron function in the central nervous system. Niacin is best known for its ability to mobilize fat from cells into the blood. This is crucial for certain detox programs that use niacin to substitute "clean" fat for "dirty" fat-holding poisons, such as heavy metals, pesticides, and solvents (see Niacin Detox Saunas in Chapter 9).

The richest food sources of vitamin B_3 include beef liver, brewer's yeast, broccoli, carrots, cheese, eggs, fish, milk, peanuts, pork, potatoes, tomatoes, and wheat germ. Whole wheat products are also good sources.

The many positive effects of vitamin B_3 on memory include the following:

- Regulates blood flow in memory tissue.

- Aids in energy production in neurons.

- Soothes outbursts in certain mental conditions.

- Strengthens GABA (gamma aminobutyric acid), a neurotransmitter that soothes neurons.

- Helps regulate blood glucose.

Recommended Dosage

Take 100 to 200 milligrams of vitamin B_3 daily with meals.

Cautionary note: As vitamin B_3 can cause a niacin "flush"—a temporary, usually harmless skin rash accompanied by slight tingling sensation—it is best to take this vitamin with meals, and preferably with yogurt. If skin flushing is a problem, try inositol hexaniacinate, a special form of niacin that is better tolerated by the body and works as well as the standard form. Do not take "time-released" niacin, which, when taken over time, may harm the liver.

Vitamin B_6 (Pyridoxine)

This very important vitamin affects several hundred chemical reactions in the brain, liver, arteries, and almost all other parts of the body. Studies indicate that most people get only about 50 percent of the required amount of B_6 for good body function. While vitamin B_6 helps trigger the production of important neurotransmitters in memory tissue, shortages allow the buildup of homocysteine, which harms the inner lining of the brain's arteries. Generally, after age forty, 25 percent more vitamin B_6 is needed than ever before.

While all foods contain some vitamin B_6, the following foods have the highest amounts: blackstrap molasses, brewer's yeast, carrots, chicken, eggs, fish, legumes, meat (especially organ meats), spinach, wheat germ, and whole grains.

Vitamin B_6 has a number of positive effects on the memory body, including the following:

- Helps supply fuel to memory neurons and other brain tissue.

- Is involved in many chemical reactions in the brain that support memory.

- Influences endocrine function in the brain.

Recommended Dosage

Take 50 milligrams of vitamin B_6 two times daily.

Cautionary note: Too much vitamin B_6 can deplete a number of other B vitamins, so always take it in balanced amounts. Vitamin B_6 is diminished by too much choline supplementation, and is neutralized by alcohol, caffeine, radiation, and cigarette smoke.

Vitamin B_{12} (Cyanocobalamin)

Vitamin B_{12} is linked to the production of acetylcholine—an important neurotransmitter that assists in memory and learning (see page 112). Helpful in preventing depression in the elderly, vitamin B_{12} is the only vitamin to have important minerals in its makeup. As vitamin B_{12} has limited absorption through the tiny blood vessels in the digestive tract, taking it with calcium will help improve its absorption. Also, be aware that the trace mineral boron is needed to aid in the absorption of calcium. Magnesium is also needed to prevent calcium from clogging blood vessels.

The largest amounts of B_{12} are found in brewer's yeast, clams, eggs, meats—especially pork, beef liver, and kidneys—mackerel, milk and other dairy products, and seafood.

Vitamin B_{12} has a number of positive effects on the memory body, including the following:

- Helps make and reactivate red blood cells. This increases the probability that memory neurons in the brain will get enough oxygen and more complete sugar metabolism to energize the movement of message information.

- Strengthens neurotransmitters.

- Builds up the nervous system, arming it against stress.

- Increases concentration.

- Helps protect arteries in the brain by metabolizing homocysteine.

Recommended Dosage

Take 400 to 1,000 micrograms of vitamin B_{12} each day. In addition to capsules and tablets, vitamin B_{12} also comes in lozenges, which are placed under the tongue, and in a gel form, which is inserted into the nose with an applicator and absorbed through the nasal passages. Intramuscular injections are also available and recommended for those with critical vitamin B_{12} deficiency. For maximum efficiency, B_{12} supplements should be accompanied by 400 micrograms of folic acid.

Cautionary note: Those with overactive or underactive thyroids may have trouble with B_{12} absorption; it is important to take the proper thyroid supplement. When taking boron to promote calcium absorption, take no more than 3 milligrams a day. Boron in high concentrations can be harmful to memory neurons. Also note that large amounts of vitamin C will wash B_{12} from the body.

Vitamin E

Because memory tissue is so energy intensive and requires nearly a quarter of all the oxygen coming into the body, the chance for free radical damage there is great. Vitamin E helps neutralize the destructive force of lone oxygen radicals that are created by the great energy needs for moving and storing memory in brain cells. While neuronal tissue uses catalase, superoxide dismutase, and glutathione peroxidase to quench free radicals, these three protective enzymes are in short supply. This is why memory neurons need the extra antioxidant power of vitamins E and C. While vitamin C occurs in large quantities in the cerebral tissue, vitamin E levels are not as plentiful.

Vitamin E passes through the blood-brain barrier with ease, making it an excellent protector of memory cells. It is also believed to help stop free radical damage and neuron loss in the substantia nigra—the nerve cluster associated with Parkinson's disease. When 70 percent of the cells in this area disappear, tremors of the hands and feet become noticeable. Vitamin E may be one of the most important supplements to help fight Parkinson's disease. If you consume a lot of canned or processed foods, or eat a lot of fast foods, vitamin E might offer some protection against the harmful flavor enhancers typically used in such products.

Rich sources of vitamin E include brown rice, eggs, legumes, nuts, milk, oatmeal, organ meats, seeds, soybeans, wheat, wheat germ, and whole grains. Dark green leafy vegetables like kale, mustard greens, and Swiss chard are also good sources.

Vitamin E has a number of positive effects on memory, including the following:

- Passes through the blood-brain barrier with ease to help eliminate free radicals where they do the most damage inside neurons.

- Helps safeguard neurons following a stroke.

- Helps reduce blood inflammation from neurotoxins, allergic responses, or infections.

- May help slow the progression of Parkinson's disease if taken as part of a memory supplement program.

- Reduces the spoilage of beneficial omega-3 fatty acids.

Recommended Dosage

Take 400 to 800 international units of vitamin E daily. Some doctors recommend more for smokers and persons living in cities with high smog levels. There is no difference in the absorption rates between fat-soluble and water-soluble vitamin E. Fat-soluble vitamin E is less expensive, however.

Cautionary note: *Those with diabetes, rheumatic heart disease, or an overactive thyroid, as well as those taking anticoagulants (blood thinners) should not take more than the recommended dose of vitamin E.*

Zinc

Even small shortages of zinc can impede concentration levels and memory processing. Experts believe that only 10 percent of the population gets enough of this mineral. Researchers believe zinc deficiency could be involved in the onset of severe memory loss. Those with Alzheimer's disease typically show low levels of zinc in memory tissue and cerebrospinal fluids. One Alzheimer's study noted that, during zinc supplementation, 80 percent of the subjects improved in communication skills, social contact with others, sentence comprehension, and recall.

Zinc, a free radical fighter, is a constituent of many vital enzymes, including the antioxidant superoxide dismutase (SOD). Sufficient intake of zinc is also necessary in maintaining the proper concentration of vitamin E in the blood. It is also helpful in increasing the absorption of vitamin A.

Brewer's yeast, egg yolks, fish, lamb, legumes, liver, mushrooms, oysters, poultry, soybeans, and sunflower seeds are rich sources of zinc. Whole grains are other good sources.

Zinc offers a number of positive effects on the memory body, including the following:

- Increases memory recall and visual patterns.

- Improves short-term memory.

- Increases attention span because it supports neuron energy needs.

- Helps reduce lead levels from smog pollution and other sources in memory tissue.

- Brings dramatic immune function response to older people.

Recommended Dosage

Take 15 to 20 milligrams of zinc a day. Men can take up to 60 milligrams a day, while women can take a maximum of 45 milligrams.

Cautionary note: Never take more than 100 milligrams of zinc in a day. While doses under 100 milligrams aid in boosting the immune system, doses higher than 100 can depress it. Too much zinc can lead to copper and iron deficiencies. While zinc has the least toxicity among the trace minerals, excessive doses taken for long periods of time can actually weaken the immune system. When taking zinc with an iron supplement, be sure to take them at different times. Taken together, these two minerals interfere with each other's activity. Select a reliable multi-mineral supplement.

BUYING "SMART" NUTRIENTS

The way supplemental vitamins, enzymes, amino acids, and minerals are processed is a crucial factor in their efficiency. Often, a person will read an article in a health magazine that recommends various supplements for a specific health problem, then run to a local discount pharmacy and buy a round of the suggested products—often the cheapest ones available. Not a wise move. When it comes to supplements, cheap often translates into ineffective. Such products can contain low concentrations of the important elements and high levels of additives. Poor processing is another likely possibility. It is important to consider quality control and production methods before you buy memory supplements. When it comes to your brain, buy only the highest quality supplements.

Importance of Plant Harvesting

The time of year a plant or herb is harvested is crucial for maximum potency. Botanical effectiveness ranges from 10 to 90 percent. Ideally, plants should be at full maturity when harvested, but not on the wane. Some are best collected in the fall, others in the spring. Harvesting procedures can differ widely also. It takes training and skill to know the variations for each plant. In some cases, extractions from a plant's root are most effective, while the stem, fruit, or leaves of other plants contain the best "medicine." As a rule of thumb, most plant or herbal ingredients should be harvested only a few weeks before they are processed.

Quality Control and Supplement Sources

Considerable skill and experience is necessary in understanding the wide variety and number of plant structures. Consumers may get "lost" in trying to verify what is really inside a supplement. Dr. Dan Mowrey, President of American Phytotherapy Research Laboratory of Salt Lake City, Utah, urges consumers to check for at least 24 percent potency in some herbal extracts like ginkgo biloba. It is one thing to indicate what a liquid or capsule contains, but what good is that knowledge if you don't know the potency? If you do not have access to a licensed nutritionist or herbalist, check your local library or bookstore for specialized information about certain plants.

Become an educated consumer. Learn as much as you can about individual supplements. What are the sources of the components in multiple vitamins or glandular products? When was the plant grown? When was it harvested? Echinacea—an herb commonly used to boost the immune system—that has been sitting on a warehouse shelf for three years won't be as potent as one harvested in the same year it is sold. For full potency, this herb should be only a few weeks old when harvested. Such "freshness" can be costly, however, with suppliers charging supplement companies more for an herb that is harvested during its botanical peak. But remember, you will be paying for quality.

Ginseng—another popular immune-enhancing herb—varies in strength and effectiveness according to where it is grown. Although some varieties of Chinese and Korean ginseng are good quality, American ginseng is considered superior. Or consider bilberry. Rich in anthocyanidins, this blueberry-like plant was a favorite among British pilots during World War II because it supposedly improved night vision. Bilberry supplements manufactured in Scandinavia are prescribed by doctors throughout Europe for people who suffer with broken veins and other vascular problems. Species of bilberry grown in the United States, however, lack the vascular-enhancing qualities found in the Scandinavian variety.

With some supplements, such as essential fatty acids (especially fish oils) and certain herbal preparations, look for third-party certification to be sure the product contains the percentage and exact substance stated on the container. A third party is generally an agency or an outside group of qualified people who examine the supplement, check its authenticity, and agree the product meets its advertised claims. Such a practice offers consumers more assurance that the product contains what is stated on the label.

Finding the Best Supplement Companies

It is important for users of supplements to understand that there are thirty to forty steps in the proper processing of most nutritional support products. A number of companies follow some but not all of the proper procedures, while others follow none. You cannot expect full benefit from a supplement if it was not manufactured using high standards. Of course, fewer processing steps cost less, bringing a higher profit return to manufacturers.

Don't be fooled by fancy containers or enticing labels. Some of the best supplements are packaged in containers with simple labels. Remember, you are not buying a label; it's what's in the container that counts. Try to avoid mass-produced health products. Smaller specialty companies that manufacture supplements only are the best choices. Keep in mind that higher quality products may be more costly, but they are likely to be more effective, as well. And remember, your memory is worth it.

Of the thousands of companies who sell nutritional supplements, only about 200 are believed to maintain the standard just described. Some of these companies, who have proven their reliability over time, include Progressive Research Laboratories, Inc., Thorne Research, Allergy Research Group, Cardiovascular Research, Ltd., and Standard Process. Other reputable companies include Atrium, Bezwecken, McZand Herbals, Metagenics, Molecular Biologics, Nutri West, Pure Encapsulation, Systemic Formula,

Tyler, and Tyson. These companies have spared no expense re-searching the best production methods of vitamins, glandulars, enzymes, and minerals for the best delivery into the bloodstream. In addition to manufacturing supplements, some of these compa-nies conduct their own supplement research as well. Always look for these brand names.

In certain areas, most of these brand-name products are avail-able only through health-care practitioners or specialized homeo-pathic pharmacies, many of which provide mail order service. Although homeopathic pharmacies are growing in number throughout the country, they can be difficult to locate. For your convenience, we have included a number of these pharmacies in the Resource List, beginning on page 199.

Buying Supplements Abroad

We do not recommend purchasing nutritional supplements from other countries for a number of reasons. For one thing, there are no guarantees on shipment delivery even if you have sent the appro-priate payment. Nor is it easy to check the source of the raw mate-rials used for the products. It is also impossible to check the way in which the supplements have been processed, as well as the clean-liness of the processing conditions. All product claims must be taken on faith.

Many high-quality products are available here in the United States. It is not necessary to search outside the country for them.

IN SUMMARY

If you have begun to experience memory loss, the time is right to start taking "smart" nutrients. Many of these substances are pow-erful antioxidants, others assist message transmission. Memory operates on electrical and chemical energy. Mineral electrolytes, enzymes, amino acids, fats, and vitamins are required to create the cellular electricity for memory within neurons, just they are need-ed to produce the chemical force to help memory jump the synap-tic gap between neurons.

Without these building blocks, your ability to process informa-tion will be weakened. The smart nutrients suggested in this chap-ter will help maintain the electrical and chemical forces in memory tissue, replenish neurotransmitter supplies, and support cerebrospinal fluids in the cerebrum. Such additions encourage good neuronal health and a return to normal memory. Make memory restoration part of your supplement plan from now on.

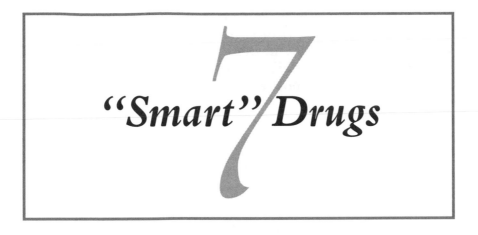

"Smart" Drugs

"It's never too late to be what you might have been."

—George Eliot

When explorer Ponce de Leon sailed to the Americas looking for the fountain of youth, he was searching for an anti-aging substance that would keep his mind sharp and his body young and virile. Today, people still yearn for this desire to maintain youth. They want to think fast, stay sharp, and be healthy. During the next ten years, 50 million American men and women will be entering their late forties and early fifties. A recent survey showed that the majority of those over fifty have a fear of age-associated memory loss. Even young college students are in constant search for better memory and sharper mental performance. As a result, cognitive enhancement has become the tenth largest subject of pharmaceutical research.

Leading pharmaceutical companies throughout the world are investing millions of research dollars into developing products that prevent memory loss. Within a few years, pharmaceuticals may be available to stop memory loss altogether with complete safety. To date, there are drugs available for improving circulation, curbing depression, and enhancing learning. Commonly known as "smart" drugs, these substances are known to scientists as *nootropics*—an ancient Greek term that means "acting on the mind." Smart drugs are often derivatives of the same neurotransmitters and support chemicals needed by your memory tissue to function. The search for the right smart drug is a search for better memory, a sharper mind, the ability to think clearly, and the capability to solve problems. No one wants to lose these functions. Smart drug research strives to support the mind in all of its cognitive and memory activities.

A WORD OF WARNING

Results from the early testing of smart drugs have excited pharmaceutical companies all over the world. Improved memory, alertness, and better ability to solve problems are some of the results smart drugs have had on lab animals. In addition, hundreds of people are reportedly taking nootropics with good results and very few side effects. But it is important for you to know that these drugs are controversial. And it is strongly recommended that smart drugs be considered only by those with serious memory problems.

Because the U.S. Food and Drug Administration (FDA) feels insufficient research has gone into the production of most nootropics, very few have been given approval for prescription or over-the-counter availability. In fact, the FDA points out that many of these drugs are manufactured outside the country and often "do not meet the quality control standards accepted in this country" and enforced by their office. The FDA is also concerned that Americans may be at risk if they take excessive doses of even ordinary vitamins, minerals, and amino acids that are manufactured outside the United States.

A number of smart drugs can be purchased from international sources through the mail. Be aware, however, that purchasing drugs manufactured in countries outside the United States lends itself to a variety of problems. For starters, consumers have reportedly sent orders for the drugs along with payment, but have failed to receive any product. More important, however, is the fact that there are no product quality guarantees. In addition, finding a doctor who has had experience with these substances can be difficult. For a listing of reputable companies who sell smart drugs outside the United States, see the Resource List beginning on page 199.

Probably the most important thing to consider, however, is that while short-term studies with lab animals have shown phenomenal improvement in mental capabilities, no one knows exactly what the long-term effects of these drugs might be. Limited studies with mice have shown that some of the positive cognitive-enhancing effects of smart drugs can be passed on to offspring. However, as these drugs are relatively new, there is much that is still unknown about them—specifically any long-term negative effects. What if smart drugs cause permanent changes of a negative nature that can be passed on from one generation to the next? Keep these issues in mind as you read this chapter.

Also, be aware that dosages for nootropic drugs are based on individual considerations, such as body weight, age, and overall allergic response. Some individuals may need more, while others require fewer concentrations of these smart drugs for true effectiveness. In addition, taking smaller amounts of certain nootropics may produce optimal results, while taking more of another type may bring positive memory change.

For all of these reasons, it is important to be cautious in your decision to take smart drugs. If you are still interested, however, it is very strongly recommended that you do so only under the guidance of a qualified health-care provider. This expert should have extensive knowledge of or be willing to learn about the qualities and quirks of the various "memory enhancing" drugs; it should be someone who will help you decide your own particular needs.

SMART DRUGS FROM A TO Z

The following pharmaceuticals have been shown to have positive effects on memory improvement. While some of these drugs have been approved by the FDA and are available by prescription, others are found outside the United States only. Once again, it cannot be stressed strongly enough that if you take any of the following smart drugs, do so only under the watchful eye of your doctor, who will help you obtain the best nootropic for your individual needs.

Aniracetam

With a chemical structure very close to piracetam (page 153), aniracetam has been documented in human tests to help men and women score better on memory and IQ tests. In a study of sixty patients in a geriatric nursing home, aniracetam showed revitalizing effects in the subjects' memory function. When compared with piracetam—the "grandfather of smart drugs"—aniracetam seems to treat more cognitive lapses associated with aging than piracetam.

In tests on laboratory animals, aniracetam demonstrated a "protective effect" on neuronal tissue. Still, scientists are not sure how this smart drug works in learning and memory tissue. Aniracetam does not appear to have an effect on the brain's main neurotransmitters: GABA, the catecholamines, serotonin, or acetylcholine. Considered an experimental cognitive substance, aniracetam has not yet been approved in the United States or abroad. As it is still in its testing stages, aniracetam cannot be prescribed by U.S. doctors or purchased through overseas mail.

Cautionary note: Aniracetam has not been tested extensively in humans. The U.S. patent is held by Hoffman-LaRoche, but they have turned the rights over to several foreign producers. It remains to be seen if aniracetam will be produced over-the-counter for worldwide sale.

Centrophenoxine

Centrophenoxine is said to increase the life span of test animals by one third when compared to a control group of animals who did not receive it. Studies conducted by a number of drug companies indicate that centrophenoxine improves learning ability, possibly due to the reduction of lipofuscin deposits in neuronal tissue. Lipofuscin deposits (brown spots) are signs of free radical damage and are associated with aging. Some researches even claim that centrophenoxine repairs damaged or weak synaptic connections between neurons. However, we suspect some other unknown mechanism is at work here, because lipofuscin is found in large amounts in normal, older people who have no memory loss.

When chemically active in the body, centrophenoxine breaks down into the memory enhancer DMAE, which, in itself, can have a positive effect on the nervous system. Its main value may be in helping cells get and use more oxygen, particularly in areas where there is tissue damage from a stroke, ruptured blood supply, atherosclerotic dementia, or angina. While it is unlikely that this drug is effective in treating advanced cases of memory loss characteristic in Alzheimer's disease, it may reduce some symptoms of mild memory loss. Trade names of centrophenoxine include: Analux, Brenal, Cerebon, Lucidril, Lutiaron, Marucotol, Mecloxate, Proseryl, and Telucidone. Presently, it is available in Mexico.

Cautionary note: Centrophenoxine should never be used by anyone who suffers from severe hypertension or convulsions. Nor should it be taken by pregnant or nursing women. Possible side effects include depression, motion sickness, hyperactivity, and drowsiness.

Deprenyl

Deprenyl is considered an anti-aging drug because it has increased life span and cognitive activity in test animals by 30 to 40 percent. Developed at Semmelweis University in Hungary by Dr. Jozsef Knoll, deprenyl is used throughout Europe as a treatment for Alzheimer's disease.

In one study, tests among ten Alzheimer's patients in Italy showed that deprenyl increases attention span and memory recall activity. Even the ability to acquire and process information improved among these patients. Some subjects noticed that deprenyl also increased their short-term and long-term memory, as well as their concentration, attention span, and verbal ability to put sentences together.

In the United States, deprenyl is typically used to treat Parkinson's disease because it seems to protect dopamine—an important neurotransmitter that regulates muscle control and elevates mood. In one study, deprenyl "rescued" 69 percent of the memory cells in mice who were deliberately given a memory-destroying neurotoxin. Deprenyl decreases high amounts of monoamine oxidase-B (MAO-B), an enzyme that gobbles up dopamine. Psychiatrist J. John Mann, M.D. of the University of Pittsburgh, found that deprenyl is three times more effective than a placebo in fighting depression.

Parkinson's disease patients show a destruction of dopamine-producing neurons in the brain. The drug levodopa (L-dopa) was developed to help protect dopamine by limiting the excessive production of the enzyme that removes this neurotransmitter from the body. Unfortunately, the effectiveness of L-dopa wears off with time, and some evidence exists that it may be toxic to memory neurons. In tests done at the University of Virginia Medical School, neuroscientists found that rats treated with L-dopa had high levels of free radical formation and an energy production slowdown in dopamine-producing neurons. Since deprenyl appears to lack negative side effects, it is increasingly being used to replace L-dopa.

A study in Finland compared neuronal tissue from Parkinson's disease victims who had taken deprenyl and L-dopa together, with the tissue of those who had been given L-dopa alone. Patients who had taken only L-dopa had a much greater neuronal loss in the substantia nigra, where dopamine is made, than did the group that had taken both deprenyl and L-dopa together.

When this discovery was made, many doctors began giving deprenyl together with L-dopa to offer more protection to their Parkinson's patients. But then some troubling evidence about deprenyl began to surface. A British study of more than 500 Parkinson's victims showed a 60 percent higher death rate in patients who were given both drugs compared to those patients given L-dopa alone. Severe problems with motion and movement were also noted in those taking both drugs.

This is an example of the possible danger of taking combinations of nootropic drugs. While the manufacturers may claim that smart drugs are not toxic, they also agree that broad-based human studies using combinations of smart drugs are limited. Use extreme caution when combining nootropic drugs.

Those with severe memory loss may want to try a drug like deprenyl. But please do so only under a doctor's professional guidance. Deprenyl is available in the United States by prescription only.

Cautionary note: *A hypertensive reaction is likely to occur if you are taking deprenyl as an MAO-B inhibitor and consume tyramine-rich foods such as beans, chicken liver, cheese, and red wine. Pharmaceutical companies claim this reaction does not occur in those taking deprenyl to fight Parkinson's disease. If you have a tendency toward allergic responses, you still might wish to avoid such foods when taking deprenyl. Also avoid the free-form amino acids phenylalanine, tyrosine, and tryptophan, which are found in certain foods like red wine, herring, and turkey.*

Do not combine deprenyl with L-dopa. And do not buy deprenyl from a country outside the United States, even if it is less expensive.

Fipexide

Fipexide, which has a small dopamine-increasing tendency, has shown improved cognitive performance in elderly patients with severe memory disorders. In one study that involved forty patients, fipexide decreased the time the subjects needed to finish a task by an average of 22 percent. Errors were decreased by 46 percent. Test animals given fipexide showed increased memory for task learning.

Not available in the United States, fipexide is found in Thailand, Japan, Italy, Spain, Belgium, England, Canada, and Mexico.

Cautionary note: As broad-based field studies and experimental research are limited for Fipexide, it may not be a very wise choice. However, if you do take it, be sure to stop immediately at the first sign of hypertension, headache, dizziness, nausea, or any other unusual symptoms.

Gerovital (H3)

Sometimes, a wonderful discovery can come about as a fruitful surprise, as Dr. Ana Aslan found out at her Romanian geriatric clinic in the 1940s. She had been treating the painful joints of arthritis patients with injections of procaine, a local anesthetic. After years of administering this treatment, Dr. Aslan noticed that her patients, in addition to being helped for their arthritis symptoms, showed marked improvement in memory, increased feelings of happiness, and raised energy levels.

Dr. Aslan found that by combining procaine with other substances—vitamin B_6, mesoinositol, potassium metabisulfite, and glutamic acid—the effects were even more impressive on aging. Dr. Aslan's research allowed her to perfect her product—called Gerovital (H3).

An effective antidepressant for long-term emotional problems, Gerovital slows down the overproduction of monoamine oxidase, which tends to gobble up needed neurotransmitters like dopamine, serotonin, and norepinephrine. This may account for the energy and mood improvement reported by those who take it. Gerovital also claims to help memory cells use oxygen more effectively in the elderly.

Although Gerovital cannot be obtained in the United States, a similar product called Gero-Vita (G.H.3) is available. Containing metabolites of procaine, Gero-Vita claims to produce the same effects as Gerovital. To purchase this product, contact Gero Vita International, 6021 Yonge Street, Department 7126E, Toronto, Ontario, 3W2, Canada; 1–800–694–8366.

Cautionary note: Gerovital has no known toxic side effects. In rare instances, it may produce allergic reactions, such as skin rashes, headaches, and changes in stool patterns.

Hydergine

Much research has gone into Hydergine, a smart drug that supports energy production in the mitochondria of memory cells. It
keeps this metabolic activity from falling below 50 percent of the
levels found in young, healthy adults—the level where senile
dementia begins to raise its head. Advocates of hydergine say it
stimulates protein synthesis, encouraging dendrite connections
with other memory cells. It appears to aid in improved thinking
functions, faster responses, and more positive moods and attitudes. Hydergine also helps older people sleep better and, of
course, it improves memory.

In animal studies, Hydergine has been shown to increase neuron cell energy activity by 25 to 30 percent, and it appears to support neuron "plasticity" by increasing the dendrite connections between memory cells during learning. Human studies have demonstrated that Hydergine helps men and women score better on tests
that evaluate mental alertness, mood, clarity of thought, and general ease of cognitive thinking. It is believed that Hydergine limits
free-radical activity and helps remove lipofuscin (age pigment) in
memory tissue. It also appears to reduce tinnitus (ringing in the
ears) and dizziness. Hydergine is available in Europe and the
United States by prescription only.

*Cautionary note: Although Hydergine is available in the United States,
many doctors are unfamiliar with its cognitive effects. If you combine
Hydergine with piracetam, cut the dose of each in half to avoid a reverse
effect on all measures. More is not better here, so try smaller doses if
using both drugs. Hydergine may cause nausea, headache, or stomach
upset if the dosage is too large.*

Idebenone

Idebenone, an antioxidant that helps reduce stroke damage in
memory tissue, is related to coenzyme Q_{10} (CoQ_{10}). Unlike CoQ_{10},
idebenone does not tend to metabolize itself into a highly reactive
free radical. In laboratory tests, idebenone has been found to shield
animals from memory loss by increasing levels of oxygen in the
blood. It also protects memory neurons from low levels of serotonin and the molecules that break down or diminish the neurotransmitter acetylcholine. In humans, low serotonin levels have
been linked to bad temper, impulsiveness, and harsh physical
behavior. Idebenone is available in Japan by prescription only.

Cautionary note: Few scientific double-blind studies have been done on idebenone outside the pharmaceutical industry.

Milacemide

Glycine is an amino acid that activates the long-term memory switches known as the N-methyl-D-aspartate (NMDA) complex. The problem is that glycine levels can fall off with age. Glycine supplements are not the answer because they do not pass through the blood-brain barrier easily. On the other hand, drug companies claim that milacemide passes through the blood-brain barrier, where it changes first into glycinamide and then into glycine. Substances that support NMDA activity also support learning. Since glycine acts as a light switch for the NMDA receptors that call up long-term memory, milacemide may have the ability to activate long-term memory that has been lost through general aging or excessive free radical damage to memory neurons.

More nondrug company-sponsored studies must be conducted to confirm whether or not milacemide truly can pass through the blood-brain barrier and then be broken down into the smaller glycine that triggers long-term memory. So far, milacemide has not helped Alzheimer's victims in test studies. Nor does it have a therapeutic effect on the treatment of schizophrenics. But milacemide may support memory tissue in normal healthy people. Since drug companies need to prove that a substance can treat a disease, milacemide could languish on the shelf.

Although milacemide is not presently available in the United States, know that you can purchase magnesium glycinate in health food stores. Magnesium glycinate is an alternative memory supplement that is used to increase your body supply of glycine.

Cautionary note: Keep in mind that most milacemide studies have been conducted on animals. Those studies involving Alzheimer's patients by drug companies have shown this smart drug to display little toxicity. Diarrhea and nausea are possible side effects. Never use milacemide with an MAO-B inhibitor such as deprenyl.

Nimodipine

The regulation of calcium in memory neurons is important. Too much calcium burns out dendrites and axons, eventually leading to the death of the whole neuron. When a person is under stress, he or she produces high levels of cortisol, which triggers calcium to flood into neurons. The calcium is then reabsorbed naturally. When stress is constant, however, the calcium has a harder time getting reabsorbed. Eventually, the calcium will have a toxic effect on the neurons.

A calcium blocker like nimodipine helps control high levels of calcium. It has been successful in relieving migraine headaches, as well as reducing the risk of high blood pressure and congestive heart failure. Available in the United States by prescription, nimodipine is recommended to improve mental clarity and memory, particularly for those with Alzheimer's disease.

Cautionary note: Overdoses of nimodipine can cause side effects, such as headaches, rashes, breathing problems, depression, swelling or edema, diarrhea, and decreased blood pressure.

Ondansetron

As people age, memory is stored less efficiently due to lowered levels of the important neurotransmitter acetylcholine. Ondansetron, developed by Glaxo Pharmaceuticals, claims to increase acetylcholine by blocking high levels of serotonin, which suppresses acetylcholine with advancing age. Ondansetron was found to improve immediate and delayed "name-face recall" in those experiencing age-associated memory impairment. These effects appeared to hold up over a twelve-week period. Glaxo researchers say another advantage to ondansetron is that it increases acetylcholine only in the part of the brain associated with memory. If true, this means ondansetron would improve memory "without causing the side effects associated with acetylcholine release in other parts of the body."

Cautionary note: Though commonly prescribed to curb nausea after chemotherapy treatments, ondansetron can cause stomach upset, rashes, seizures, chest pain, and breathing spasms.

Oxiracetam

Compared to piracetam, only one-third the amount of oxiracetam is needed to improve memory when testing new-task learning in normal, healthy mice. Italian researchers showed that the offspring of mice given oxiracetam, were more "curious" and scored better on memory tests than the offspring of mice who never received it. This is both fascinating and troublesome because oxiracetam appears to have the ability to affect genetic transmission of learning. While at first, this may appear to be a good thing, there is also a downside—what if oxiracetam can pass on negative characteristic not yet known to the next generation? Oxiracetam also appears to decrease blood clotting in older people. This suggests some value for multi-infarct patients who want to avoid memory loss.

Presently, oxiracetam is available in Italy and Japan.

Cautionary note: Oxiracetam has been shown to be safe in daily doses of up to 2,400 milligrams.

Phenytoin (Dilantin)

An FDA-approved treatment for epilepsy found under the trade name Dilantin, phenytoin is used to treat a number of diseases, as well. As far as its effects on memory, phenytoin stabilizes electrical activity in cell membranes. Tests have shown it can improve intelligence scores on the Wechsler IQ test. Phenytoin seems to have a positive effect on long-term memory and verbal performance in both the young and the elderly. Some have found that it helps alleviate jet lag and sleeping problems, while increasing stamina. Research conducted with prison inmates showed that Dilantin normalized overly passive or violent tendencies.

The book *A Remarkable Medicine Has Been Overlooked* by Jack Dreyfus cites the positive effects of phenytoin on obsessive depression. In neurological research, phenytoin has shown an ability to restore brain hormone imbalance to youthful, normal levels that are lost as one grows older. In small doses, phenytoin increases levels of high density lipoproteins (HDLs)—the good cholesterol.

Cautionary note: Phenytoin can cause a drastic reduction in vitamin B_{12} reserves, and it can increase the need for thyroid hormone. This drug should not be used by pregnant women, or those with heart or kidney problems. High doses of phenytoin may also cause gum overgrowth.

Piracetam (Nootropil)

The "grandfather of smart drugs," piracetam is probably taken by more people to alleviate memory problems than any other smart drug. Originally brought to market by UCB Laboratories in Belgium, piracetam is available in a number of countries. It is not, however, sold in the United States. Enthusiasts claim piracetam increases memory, mental clarity and alertness, verbal ability, problem solving ability, and concentration. According to pharmaceutical literature, piracetam is similar to the amino acid pyroglutamine, and works by stimulating the nerve tracts that produce acetylcholine—the number one neurotransmitter.

Marketed to improve memory flow in people with low oxygen levels in the brain, piracetam has also been used to treat vertigo, senile dementia, sickle cell anemia, dyslexia, and stroke. Piracetam protected memory in laboratory rats when they were denied oxygen, a similar condition to that which develops in stroke victims. Pharmaceutical representatives say there is evidence that piracetam might improve the information pathway between the left and right hemispheres of the brain.

Since its arrival in the marketplace, pharmaceutical companies have produced other forms of piracetam, such as aniracetam, oxiracetam, and pramiracetam. These drugs appear to offer more benefits than piracetam at lower doses. However, piracetam continues to be a favorite with consumers and is often combined with other smart drugs and various supplements.

We urge you to use caution when taking piracetam with any other memory drug. Please do so only under the prudent advice of a doctor who is experienced in this field. If you do start adding other smart drugs to piracetam, add only one new drug at a time, and watch carefully for any negative responses.

In one study, test rodents given piracetam for two weeks had a 30 to 40 percent increase in certain memory receptors, increasing their memory storage. Biological researcher Arthur Cherkin believed a normal dose of piracetam could be made five times as strong if combined with hydergine. Other pharmaceutical-funded research has shown an increased effect in piracetam if it is taken with various combinations of DMAE, centrophenoxine, hydergine, and choline. Do not expect piracetam to help with sleep disturbances, depression, or muscular speed, as do some "smart" drugs. It brings more results in basic cognition and memory areas of dysfunction.

Cautionary note: *Rare side effects of piracetam may include gastrointestinal disturbance, headache, nausea, and insomnia.*

Pramiracetam

Developed from the piracetam molecule, pramiracetam is said to strengthen neurotransmitter functions in memory. Although lower doses than piracetam are needed, the effects of pramiracetam are estimated to be fifteen times stronger. Limited research has shown pramiracetam to be more helpful in the treatment of Alzheimer's victims than piracetam.

Also known as CI-879, pramiracetam is still in its testing stages and not yet available abroad or in the United States.

Cautionary note: Should pramiracetam become available, be cautious and monitor your physical responses carefully. To date, pharmaceutical literature indicates no known toxicity.

Propranolol Hydrochloride (Inderal)

Propranolol hydrochloride controls high blood pressure and blocks the receptor site for adrenaline, the fight-or-flight neurotransmitter. Fear and anxiety cause a rush of adrenaline which, in turn, can bring on more fear and anxiety, creating an unhealthy cycle. In addition to adrenaline, anxiety causes the release of high levels of cortisol, which triggers calcium to flood into neurons. The calcium is reabsorbed naturally. When stress is constant, however, the calcium has a harder time getting reabsorbed. Eventually, the calcium will have a toxic effect on the neurons. Propranolol hydrochloride helps control fear and stress reactions, limiting the buildup of cortisol. It is available in the United States by prescription.

Cautionary note: As propranolol hydrochloride reduces blood pressure, those with low blood pressure should avoid it. To prevent stomach upset or nausea, always take this drug with food, and never take it within two weeks of taking an MAO inhibitor. It is not advisable to take propranolol hydrochloride before a competitive event in which you need a boost of adrenaline. Others who should avoid propranolol hydrochloride include pregnant women and those with asthma, pollen allergies, tendencies toward arterial spasms, diabetes, and kidney or liver problems.

Vasopressin (Diapid)

A hormone of the posterior pituitary gland, vasopressin relieves the need to frequently urinate in those patients with diabetes insipidus, an unusual form of diabetes. Available in the United States by prescription, vasopressin is believed also to improve attention span, concentration, and memory retention, as well as short- and long-term memory. According to some individuals, vasopressin helps store large amounts of new memory information. Neurologists believe it is helpful in the storage of new memories. To help preserve your body's natural vasopressin, avoid the use of amphetamines.

Cautionary note: Vasopressin may produce nasal congestion or irritation of the nasal passages, headaches, stomach cramps, and increased bowel movements. Vasopressin should not be taken during pregnancy.

Vincamine (Oxicebral)

An extract of periwinkle, vincamine expands blood vessels, increasing blood flow to the brain. It also helps memory tissue make better use of the brain's oxygen. Presently available only in Europe, vincamine has been reported to stabilize the brain-wave patterns of seniors with memory trouble. It also helps revive memory in the alcoholic brain.

Cautionary note: Vincamine may cause stomach upset. Little research has been done on this drug to substantiate its pharmaceutical claims.

Vinpocetine

Presently unavailable in the United States, vinpocetine is manufactured in Hungary. It is a powerful memory enhancer that claims to help cerebral energy conversion by supporting circulation in tiny blood vessels. It also increases the utilization of oxygen and sugar. Those who have difficulty in verbal expression or experience an inability to coordinate movements claim vinpocetine has helped.

Gedeon Richter, a Hungarian pharmaceutical company, has funded over 100 studies on vinpocetine. These studies have indicated the drug's positive results with minimal side effects. In tests involving over 800 patients with memory loss caused by stroke, low blood flow, or low cell energy, Gedeon Richter found that vinpocetine increases blood flow specifically in the affected areas. This drug also claims to bring noticeable short-term memory improvement. Although it is a derivative of vincamine, vinpocetine appears to have fewer negative side effects and more positive benefits.

Cautionary note: Though rare, reported side effects have included dry mouth, weakness, hypotension, and rapid heartbeat.

Xanthinol Nicotinate

A form of niacin, xanthinol nicotinate is believed to treat low blood flow to memory tissue, to arteries, and to the hands and feet. One study showed that this drug brought short-term memory enhancement to people under age fifty. Those over fifty showed improved memory response time. As a vasodilator, xanthinol nicotinate has been used to lower blood cholesterol; as it passes easily through the cell wall, it is believed to increase sugar metabolism and cellular energy. Unavailable in the United States, xanthinol nicotinate is available in Europe and Canada.

Cautionary note: Be aware that extensive field studies of xanthinol nicotinate are very limited. Reported side effects include heart palpitations, heartburn, headache, and blurred vision, which generally go away over time. Manufacturers caution that those who take xanthinol nicotinate may experience a drop in blood pressure when rising from a chair or bed. Pregnant women should not take this drug, nor should those with a severe liver problem, hypotension, congestive heart failure, or a recent myocardial infarction.

IN SUMMARY

The search for a way to prevent memory loss and cognitive function is not new. During the last fifty years, there has been a big push for the development of smart drugs. Pharmaceutical companies throughout the world have been busy working toward the production of commercial products to help stop age-related memory loss.

While great strides have been made in this area, keep the following suggestions in mind when considering smart drug use. First of all, only those with severe memory problems should look into these drugs. And then, it is strongly recommended that these medications be taken only under the expertise of a qualified health care professional—one who has knowledge of nootropics. Also, remember, while some of these drugs are FDA approved, many are not. This means drugs sold outside the United States may not have undergone extensive studies or testing. Finally, and maybe most important, the long-term effects of smart drugs still remain to be seen. Hopefully, more in-depth research and more field studies will be carried out to make sure there are no long-term negative effects that will harm you or be passed on to your offspring through DNA mutations.

Be especially careful when combining smart drugs. Again, do so only under the watchful eye of a physician who has had experience with them. When taking any smart drug, either alone or in combination with others, be sure to monitor your responses. Stop taking these substances at the first sign of abnormal cognitive or physical reaction.

Smart drugs may have a more stable place in the future when more extensive clinical studies are completed to assure consumers of their safety. Given the fact that their long-range effects are unknown, it is recommended that you first consider a natural alternative instead of synthetic drugs. These nutritional supplements, which are presented in Chapter 6, are the recommended starting place.

Chelation and Oxygen Healing Therapies

*"Keep your face to the sunshine and you cannot see
the shadow."*

—Helen Keller

*I*magine yourself climbing up a steep hill with a load of rocks on your back. You would probably be straining all the way. If more stones were added, you might even slip and fall. A similar burden exists when environmental poisons enter your bloodstream through the foods you eat, the air you breathe, and the things you touch. It won't be long before these substances enter the area in your brain where memory is stored.

For a while, the blood-brain barrier offers some protection around most of your neurons, but, as discussed earlier, certain brain areas lack this special two-layer shield. Mounting evidence links the toxic entry of various poisons through these unprotected places with the disappearance of crucial neurons for memory. In fact, the accumulation of mercury, cadmium, nickel, and other heavy metals is found in excess in the memory tissue of those with Alzheimer's disease.

With over 5,000 new chemical substances entering the marketplace every year, it is hard to estimate all the possible neurotoxic contaminants that can affect the memory neurons inside your brain. Substances like formaldehyde, cleaning solvents, smog, and pesticides are linked to the free radical damage that also seems to destroy memory neurons in otherwise healthy tissue.

LIGHTENING THE BURDEN ON MEMORY TISSUE

If neurotoxins can be removed from the blood, key memory areas in the brain, especially those not protected by the blood-brain barrier, will sustain less free radical damage. Also, the blood-brain barrier's two-layer protective net will experience less attack on its cell walls. Chelation therapy is an effective treatment to help clean the neurotoxins from the blood and brain cells.

Oxygen therapies, which include hyperbaric oxygen therapy, hydrogen peroxide therapy, and ozone therapy, are used to elevate the amount of oxygen in the bloodstream. When a body is deprived of oxygen, it is more susceptible to fatigue, weakened immunity, and poor circulation.

Used in Europe, Japan, Russia, and Cuba, chelation and oxygen therapy treatments appear to assist recovery in a wide variety of illnesses. They can speed up stroke recovery time, curb inflammation, and increase oxygen availability for neurons. When memory neurons are unburdened from toxic overload, the brain has a greater probability of healing itself.

As noted in an earlier chapter, many specific forces collide in the brain to destroy memory. These include insufficient levels of oxygen, the presence of chemical neurotoxins and free radicals, poor diets that include excessive refined sugar and fats, chronic low levels of blood sugar, mold and yeast infections, parasites that lead to increased gut permeability, low neurotransmitter levels, and the buildup of fat-stored toxins and heavy metals. Any and all of these factors can contribute to the toxic brain and the demise of memory.

There is no reason for such a bad ending to memory cells. With today's knowledge and technology, you can take positive steps to curb the harmful effects that burden memory. Chelation and oxygen therapies can help achieve these means.

CHELATION THERAPY

Like a magnet that attracts iron filings, the process of chelation (pronounced *key lay' shun*) works by drawing heavy metals and other toxins from the blood. A chelating substance is slowly introduced into the patient's bloodstream as he or she sits quietly in a chair. The most common of these substances is the synthetic amino acid ethylene diamine tetraacetic acid (EDTA). EDTA offers a bonding source for heavy metals and other poisons in the blood. Once the poisons are "bound," they are expelled from the body through the urine or feces. When foreign substances are removed from the blood, the vascular structures of the body can eventually heal themselves. Inflammation is lowered and free radical damage is slowed.

When the body is young, certain enzymes and amino acids that are designed to bind metabolic waste and poisons are present. As the body ages, however, this ability is weakened. Given the increasing amounts of environmental poisons we face every day, chelation may be one of the best ways to keep such neurotoxicity from killing memory neurons.

The History of Chelation Therapy

Swiss Nobel Laureate Alfred Warner first suggested in 1893 that toxic metals in the bloodstream could be removed by some sort of binding agent. After its development in Germany in the 1930s, chelation therapy was introduced in the United States in 1948. During World War II, the chelating agent dimercaprol was used to pull arsenic from the blood of soldiers who had been sprayed with the poison gas lewisite. There was, however, a problem. Dimercaprol caused painful and irritating side effects, so its use was abandoned. In 1952, EDTA was used as a chelating agent to alleviate arterial hardening. Because EDTA exhibits no apparent negative side effects if it is slowly dripped into the blood, its use has continued. EDTA has been used successfully to pull lead and other heavy metals from the blood. It has also been effective against radiation toxicity and snake venom poisoning.

Because of its ability to clean blood and arteries, chelation has been used successfully to reverse hardening of the arteries and increase blood flow. It has also been reported to help control, and sometimes reverse, the degenerative effects of arthritis, stroke, osteoporosis, memory loss, and senility.

How Does Chelation Work?

Some have compared chelation to a "crab's claw" that reaches out and pulls heavy metals into a new, altered chemical union. Once this binding process has occurred, the once neurotoxic metals are no longer harmful to the memory neurons. They are eliminated from the body through stool or urine. When toxic levels of heavy metals and other poisons are pulled from the blood, the turn-around in a patient's life speaks for itself. Return to a normal memory has been experienced by about half of those who have undergone this treatment.

Many advocates of conventional medicine refuse to acknowledge the value of chelation for promoting cardiovascular health or memory improvement. They opt, instead, for expensive drug treatment and surgery for heart and stroke patients—treatments that often target the symptoms rather than the causes of the conditions. Yet, cardiovascular disease remains the number one killer in the United States and many other nations. Chelation, on the other hand, offers the chance to get closer to the *cause* of memory failure. It is believed to heal the vascular system through the removal of toxic metals, which harm the blood-brain barrier and cause inflammation to memory neurons.

Why Would I Need Chelation Therapy?

In addition to the constant exposure to environmental toxins in the air and water, there are a number of other reasons a body may benefit from chelation therapy. For instance, there is the increasing popularity of precooked, convenience foods. No longer do you have to spend time cooking meals from scratch when it is easier to pick something up at the corner fast food outlet, or whip up something processed. Want mashed potatoes? No peeling needed. Just tear open a little bag of dehydrated potatoes and add water. Working late? No problem. Get a bag of burgers or tacos on the way home.

Steady diets of processed or "junk" foods eventually begin to clog blood vessels with fat and cholesterol; they also add chemical toxins from flavor enhancers and other harmful food additives to the blood. Chelation therapy can help clean this sludge from the blood and blood vessels. Affecting not only the symptoms and damaging traits of arterial disease, chelation therapy has been reported to alleviate the symptoms of multi-infarct dementia and Alzheimer's disease—conditions that stem from hardening of the arteries and high concentrations of neurotoxic substances in memory tissue.

Such cellular garbage, which is held together by a pasty form of calcium, cannot be broken down easily in the body when disease conditions exist. Chelation helps remove this plaque, allowing the blood to send other waste materials to the kidneys for removal. Once this happens, the blood vessels are free to re-establish arterial flow to the brain and other body cells.

Many people over age fifty who live in large urban areas with high levels of air and water pollution can be at high risk for neurotoxicity. Chelation may be an excellent preventive step for avoiding eventual neurological damage. Also, dentists, dental hygienists, auto mechanics, plumbers, and others who are constantly exposed to heavy metals may benefit from chelation therapy. A simple hair analysis will determine toxicity levels.

Chelation cannot reverse the tissue scarring that occurs when neurons die, but it does appear to halt the breakdown of collagen structures that weaken cell membranes as it cleans toxic metals from the blood. When you stop these cellular outlaws from barreling through the blood-brain barrier, supporters of chelation believe you are helping to stop the manufacture of the neurofibrillary tangles and amyloid plaques that are characteristic of Alzheimer's disease.

Other Features of Chelation

As a person ages, the cell walls of blood vessels tend to weaken and become more permeable or "leaky." It is especially important during this time to keep arterial structures clean and free from calcium buildup. Chelation helps by dissolving this plaque.

If the blood-brain barrier has already been compromised, lowering heavy metal levels is extremely important in protecting the fragile signal stations of neuronal dendrites and axons that carry messages in memory tissue. The synaptic spaces between neurons, where memory flashes in a thousandth of a second, are also saved from destruction.

Another feature of chelation is that it locks up the calcium that carries disease-producing organisms to other parts of the body, including cancer cells that may be lying dormant for years. In cases of heavy metal poisoning, chelation also seems to activate the body's own repair mechanisms once the load on the immune system is lessened. When this happens, there tends to be a "softening" of the vascular hardening that occurs with cardiovascular disease. This means blood vessels in the brain will also be more flexible and better able to bring blood-carrying oxygen and nutrition to memory neurons.

There is no age limit for chelation therapy. People in their nineties have experienced improved mental clarity following EDTA treatments.

What Is the Cost of Chelation Treatment?

At this time, the average cost for an intravenous chelation treatment is between $75 and $100. Insurance companies do not cover this therapy for the treatment of cardiovascular problems. A growing number of doctors are hoping to show medical insurance carriers that chelation therapy will save them money in the long run.

When figuring out the cost of chelation, be sure to include charges for urine tests, which are needed to monitor kidney function during treatments. People with kidney disease should have a urine test before each chelation treatment, others should have one every third treatment. The number of chelation treatments needed will vary, depending on the condition of the patient. People with serious cardiovascular and neurovascular damage, for example, will probably require anywhere from thirty to ninety chelation treatments for best results.

Is Intravenous the Only Method Used for Chelation Treatment?

As intravenous chelation is somewhat expensive, know that certain oral vitamin chelators like magnesium, vitamin C, choline, pantothenic acid, bioflavonoids, and seaweed preparations exist and can help clean your blood vessels. However, oral chelation may take three or four years to accomplish what intravenous chelation can do in six months to a year under a doctor's supervision. Oral vitamin chelators can also be taken in conjunction with the intravenous type.

How Marsha Got Her Memory Back

At fifty-three, Marsha, a once-energetic costumer for a major Hollywood film studio, began experiencing serious short-term memory loss. After a series of costly mistakes at work, Marsha lost her job. Soon after, her long-term memory began to fail. She began to forget things like her next door neighbor's name, and how to get back home when she went out. Marsha's brother had recently read an article about chelation therapy as an aid to memory loss. After doing a little research, he found a doctor who was experienced in performing this treatment and made an appointment for Marsha to see him.

One of the first things the doctor did was order a full range of tests, including hair analysis. This analysis showed that Marsha had high levels of cadmium, nickel, mercury, and lead in her system. Also, an amino acid panel indicated that Marsha had a significant shortage of glutamine, an important neurotransmitter used by the brain to clean out waste from memory tissue.

The doctor started Marsha on a series of intravenous chelation treatments to remove the plaque deposits and heavy metals from her circulatory system. In addition, the doctor designed a memory supplement plan for her. After four weeks and twenty-four chelation treatments, there was no noticeable improvement in Marsha's memory. Discouraged, she considered dropping the treatments. The doctor, however, reassured her that in cases of moderate to advanced memory loss, more treatments were generally needed.

By the time Marsha had received a total of forty treatments, she began to experience a return to improved memory function. Twenty-five additional sessions showed a clear indication that Marsha was on the road to memory restoration. When her hair was analyzed for heavy metals a year later, the levels were reduced significantly. Chelation therapy had done its job.

To maintain the positive results of this therapy, many chelation practitioners recommend that patients continue receiving one treatment each month. This is especially encouraged for those who do not make any positive changes in their lifestyle.

What Caused Marsha's Toxic Buildup?

When Marsha was born, she was not genetically predisposed to allergies. But by the time she was twelve, Marsha had been exposed to the nickel in her dental braces, the aluminum from the cookware her mother used, and the mercury in her dental amalgams. During much of Marsha's youth, her family's fruit orchards were sprayed with DDT until it was banned in the 1970s. When Marsha's family moved to Los Angeles, they settled in an area near several large oil refineries. This exposed them to air that was filled with petrochemical waste materials and local water supplies that were polluted with heavy metals. In the 1960s, few people were aware of the dangers caused by toxic industrial waste.

As heavy metals like cadmium, nickel, aluminum, mercury, and lead accumulated in her blood, Marsha's body defenses were under constant pressure to fight off these harmful substances, creating an allergic response known as an *immune complex*. When she was young, Marsha's body produced enough enzymes to dissolve and excrete these toxins from her body. But as time passed and her blood continued to be exposed to more and more environmental poisons, Marsha's immune system became exhausted. In addition, Marsha's eating habits were a disaster. Processed and fast foods along with sugar-laden soft drinks were the mainstays of her diet. She never ate enough enzyme-rich fresh raw fruits and vegetables, which her body needed to clean the toxic overload. Soon, Marsha's immune defenses weakened and her body was unable to get rid of the toxic buildup in her body. Her blood began to fill with immune garbage and fatty plaque materials that were no longer being broken down and eliminated.

When immune complexes were first formed by Marsha's body defenses, they circulated around in her blood. But once their number got too great, they began settling in tissue—joint cartilage or nerve tissue—causing inflammation throughout her body. When her memory tissue became inflamed, neurons began to die, resulting in memory loss. Luckily, chelation treatments were able to reduce the heavy metal overload and vascular plaque.

What Will My Doctor Say About Chelation?

Healing the body from chelation is not a mainstream therapy in the allopathic or traditional medical world. Be prepared for any number of reactions from your doctor, ranging from encouragement to dismissal. Some physicians may not know enough about chelation therapy to make an educated judgment, while others may reject it simply because it is not an accepted conventional procedure. Though there are more than 1,500 published, scientifically documented articles on chelation, controversy surrounds this treatment in traditional medical literature.

About half of the senior citizens who have undergone chelation therapy have been documented to have improved memory retention, increased IQ, and better ability to function in everyday life. According to the American College of Advancement in Medicine (ACAM), accumulated reports show that about 500,000 people around the world have had EDTA chelation therapy. As no deaths or drastic side effects have been recorded, ACAM states chelation therapy is one of the best and safest treatments for removing neurotoxicity and free radical buildup in blood and body tissue.

How Long Does a Treatment Last?

During chelation treatment, EDTA is injected drop by drop into a vein over a ninety minute to three hour period. Doctors offering EDTA chelation usually have a comfortable chair with arm rests and little writing panels so that you can read or write letters during the EDTA drip. You must be prepared to sit still, so wear comfortable clothing and bring something to do or read.

Are There Precautions for Chelation Therapy?

As long as your doctor is board-certified in chelation and follows the suggested protocol developed by the American College of Advancements in Medicine, you should experience no problems with chelation therapy. Keep the following points in mind:

- Never encourage a doctor to speed up the intravenous infusion of EDTA into your blood. The dosage and time allotted for the drip is decided on an individual basis.

- Although most people have no reactions to the drip, occasionally the skin at the site of the needle may become warm or itchy. If this causes discomfort, the doctor will simply find another vein.

- Wait for at least forty-eight hours between treatments. Your kidneys need time to rest from their excretion of chelating agents before the next treatment.

- To avoid the possibility of allergic response to the particular chelator being infused in your blood, consider an NAET treatment for this purpose. These treatments, which are detailed in Chapter 9, remove the blockages caused by immune responses, allergies, emotional stress, and chemical sensitivities.

- Those with kidney problems should have their creatinine levels checked before each chelation treatment. Removed by the kidneys, creatinine is a metabolic waste product. High levels of creatinine indicate the EDTA may cause the kidneys to overwork. If this is the case, the chelation specialist will reduce the amount of EDTA.

As long as the standard guidelines for administering chelation treatments are followed, kidney damage should not be a concern. No cases of kidney damage have ever been recorded from chelation as long as these guidelines are followed. In fact, many doctors have noted that kidney function actually improves after a series of EDTA intravenous administrations. But allergic response makes EDTA monitoring a necessary step.

How Can I Contact a Certified Chelating Physician?

To find a certified chelation practitioner in your area, contact one of the following organizations:

American Board of Chelation
  Therapy
1407 North Wells Street
Chicago, IL 60610
1–800–356–2228

American College for Advancement
  in Medicine (ACAM)
PO Box 3427
Laguna Hills, CA 92654
1–800–532–3688

The American Board of Chelation Therapy wrote the chelation protocol for certifying physicians who want to administer this treatment. The American College for Advancement in Medicine has an up-to-date directory of certified chelating physicians in your area.

A Final Word on Chelation Therapy

Physicians who have witnessed the success of chelation therapy in patients often say it is the ultimate anti-aging therapy for memory tissue. Just know that results will not occur overnight. Chelation therapy may require a number of treatments to improve neuron function.

OXYGEN HEALING THERAPIES

Oxygen is found everywhere on our planet. Sixty-two percent of the Earth's crust, oceans, rocks, plants, and animal life is made up of oxygen. The human body is no exception. Oxygen is essential to human life for two reasons. First, it is one of the basic building blocks of the body, making up more than 64 percent of all the cells in your bones, muscle, cartilage, and blood. Second, oxygen is necessary for certain chemical reactions in the body that result in energy production. And, of course, energy is necessary for basic bodily functions such as circulation, respiration, and digestion.

When oxygen levels fall in the body, illness can occur. Some bacteria even thrive in low levels of oxygen. Doctors have long treated illness and disease with oxygen. During World War I, for example, both Allied and German doctors used oxygen to cleanse battle wounds. Oxygen therapy also assisted human recovery during the worldwide influenza epidemic of 1917. In 1966, two-time Nobel Prize recipient Otto Warburg showed that when oxygen levels are low, cancer can get a foothold in the body and thrive. This discovery spurred renewed interest in finding ways to increase levels of cellular oxygen, particularly in the blood.

Oxygen therapies include hyperbaric oxygen therapy (HBOT), hydrogen peroxide therapy, and ozone therapy. Through oxygenation or oxidation, these therapies increase oxygen supplies in the blood and tissues.

These therapies work in a number of ways to aid memory. First of all, they strengthen the red blood cells that feed memory, and they help keep the membranes surrounding memory cells flexible for nutrient absorption. In addition, oxygen therapies help improve the body's own enzyme processes that fight brain aging. They also speed up energy production from sugar in the blood and neurons. Finally, these therapies increase oxygen levels in memory tissue.

Hyperbaric Oxygen Therapy

Hyperbaric oxygen therapy (HBOT) increases the concentration of oxygen in the blood. It is generally administered in oxygen chambers consisting of seven-foot-long acrylic tubes that are about twenty-five inches in diameter. A patient reclines on a stretcher that slides into the tube, which is then sealed. Increased concentrations of pure oxygen are administered under pressure for several hours. Breathing pure oxygen while in this pressurized chamber introduces more oxygen into the body's tissues and blood. Some newer chambers can accommodate several people at once. They are larger and more comfortable than the single tubes, which are confining.

Traditionally, hyperbaric oxygen treatments have been used in the United States to treat scuba divers who rise too quickly from deep waters. These divers experience dangerous air embolisms and decompression sickness. In recent years, HBOT has been used to treat a number of illnesses and conditions including strokes, brain and nerve disorders, burns, poisonings, and circulatory problems.

Considered safe, HBOT provides extra oxygen for blood and body tissues with virtually no harmful or dangerous side effects. The only reported short-term discomfort in a few cases has been minor sinus or ear pressure, similar to what one may experience when ascending or descending in an airplane. HBOT should not be used by those with a pneumothorax—a rare condition in which air is present in the chest cavity that surrounds the lung. It is a good idea for most patients to have a chest x-ray before undergoing HBOT. Pregnant women should not undergo hyperbaric oxygen therapy, except in the case of carbon monoxide poisoning. In such an instance, this can be a life-saving therapy for the unborn child.

The sooner a person who can benefit from oxygen therapy gets to a hyperbaric unit, the sooner healing can begin. In some stroke cases, for instance, the patient can minimize damage to memory cells if oxygen is supplied within two to three hours following the stroke. For this reason, it is wise to find out where these chambers are located in your area, especially if you are over fifty-five and prone to strokes or other cardiovascular problems. For further information, contact the Ocean Hyperbaric Center, 4001 North Ocean Drive, Suite 105, Lauderdale-by-the Sea, Florida, 33308, 1–954–771–4000; or the Yutsis Center for Integrative Medicine, 6413 Bay Parkway, Brooklyn, New York, 1–718–621–0900. For the quarterly journal *Undersea and Hyperbaric Medicine*, contact the Undersea and Hyperbaric Medical Society (UHMS), 10531 Metropolitan Avenue, Kensington, Maryland, 20895–2627, 1–301–942–2980.

Hydrogen Peroxide Therapy

Hydrogen peroxide therapy is another oxygen treatment that can be used to heal memory tissue by removing plaque buildup in the arteries and increasing blood flow to the brain. Naturally occurring in the body, hydrogen peroxide is necessary for proper functioning of the immune system. It helps stimulate production of the body's infection-fighting white blood cells. Hydrogen peroxide also works as a hormone regulator, and has been shown to be effective in fighting infections and treating allergies, depression, chronic fatigue syndrome, vascular headaches, Parkinson's disease, and Alzheimer's disease.

Studies performed during the 1960s at Baylor University Medical Center in Texas concluded that hydrogen peroxide injections produce the same curative result as hyperbaric oxygen therapy. It appears to have a healing effect on the blood vessel structure throughout the body, including the brain's memory tissue. The Baylor researchers reported that hydrogen peroxide relieves the violent heart contractions during myocardial ischemia. It has also been shown to clean blood vessels that are clogged with plaque.

Studies performed at New England Medical Center Hospital in Boston, Massachusetts, Upstate Medical Center in Syracuse, New York, and University of Massachusetts Medical School in Worcester, Massachusetts, showed that hydrogen peroxide seems to change the way blood thickens. This lowers the risk of clots in blood vessels throughout the body.

Hydrogen peroxide can be injected directly into muscles, joints, and soft tissues to bring healing relief to body tissue. But the method recommended most by the late Dr. Charles Farr, a doctor nominated for the Nobel Prize for his hydrogen peroxide research, is intravenous infusion. A special healing mixture of hydrogen peroxide is slowly dripped into the blood over a period of one to three hours. This method allows doctors to control the amount of hydrogen peroxide given for the best healing effect. The number of treatments needed depends on the severity of the illness.

Patients and doctors alike have worried that hydrogen peroxide might be a source of cellular aging due to free radicals. Studies have shown, however, that as long as oral iron supplements are not taken during treatment, and the hydrogen peroxide is given in the proper amounts under proper supervision, it will not form free radicals. When undergoing hydrogen peroxide treatment, drink only distilled water. Never drink tap water, which may contain minerals with oxidative properties. And because it has such powerful oxidizing effects, hydrogen peroxide should never be taken with vitamins, minerals, heparin, EDTA, amino acids, or proteins.

Although some people use hydrogen peroxide in oral or rectal treatments, we do not recommend such procedures. Taken in these forms, hydrogen peroxide may inflame the stomach or colon, possibly promoting tumor growth. Some individuals have tried therapeutic soaks in bath water to which a pint of 35 percent hydrogen peroxide has been added. There is, however, no scientific evidence that this treatment is effective for memory. Intravenous or intramuscular methods under the close supervision of a board certified practitioner are the recommended methods. (For practitioner referrals, see page 173.)

Ozone Therapy

The air we breathe contains two oxygen atoms (O_2), ozone contains three (O_3). During oxidation in the body, ozone increases the oxygen content of the blood and tissues. As a result, ozone therapy improves and accelerates wound healing while fighting fungal, bacterial, and viral infections. It also increases oxygen levels, which help increase brain energy.

Internally, this therapy involves the injection of a diluted ozone solution into veins, between joints (for arthritis or other joint problems), or into muscles. As a rectal infusion, ozone therapy is used for treating colitis and colon cancer. Ozonated water can be swabbed on the skin or used in a bath to cleanse wounds, treat burns, and heal skin infections. Topical ozonated creams and oils can be used to treat insect bites and skin wounds.

In a Cuban study, ozone therapy was used to treat cases of senile dementia in a group of elderly patients. While the therapy did not reverse memory loss, it did improve the subjects' overall quality of life. For instance, the patients exhibited increased energy and a greater ability to cope with daily life. In many cases it alleviated the symptoms of depression.

Research performed at the Medical Institute in Nizhny Novgorod, Russia, involving thirty-nine patients with severe atherosclerosis, showed ozone therapy to reduce angina attacks by nearly two-thirds. Nitroglycerine doses were lowered in the study subjects. During the ozone therapy, the patients' cholesterol blood levels dropped 48 percent while triglyceride levels decreased by more than 50 percent. The Russian doctors concluded that ozone treatment under proper medical supervision is a low-cost, effective way to deal with cardiovascular diseases.

Ozone treatments given by competent physicians may offer an excellent, early treatment for memory preservation. They can increase oxygen in memory tissue and help maintain neuron energy levels. Some experts believe ozone therapy can also help control brain inflammation due to toxic exposures that come with everyday life.

Countries worldwide use ozone therapy as a standard treatment. Since the 1950s, over 10 million ozone treatments have been given in Germany alone. In the United States, however, ozone treatment facilities are limited. Advocates in favor of these therapies believe this is because oxygen as a treatment form cannot be patented and is, therefore, not profitable for large pharmaceutical companies. Critics respond by pointing out the lack of oxygen therapy research.

How Can I Contact a Trained Oxygen Therapist?

For referrals of trained physicians in oxidative therapies, contact the International Oxidative Medicine Association (IOMA), PO Box 891954, Oklahoma City, Oklahoma, 73109, 1–405–634–1310. This association will help you locate a trained therapist in your area; however, it does not provide literature or give diagnoses.

CONCLUSION

In this chapter, you have seen how chelation and oxygen therapies can help support neuronal tissue when heavy metal concentrations are high, when stroke has occurred, or when free radical damage has wreaked havoc on the brain's memory tissue. With such knowledge, you can make your own informed choices and further investigate these treatments. One may be a good choice for you or someone you know. In the next chapter, you will learn of some other means of reducing the poisons in memory tissue.

NAET, Niacin Detox Saunas, and Fasting

"In the depth of winter, I finally learned that within me lay an invincible summer."

—Albert Camus

Science teacher Scott P. had "been there and done that" with various medical treatments for his headaches, confusion, and loss of mental focus. Whenever he expressed concern over his waning memory, he was told nothing could be done about it. Then a doctor explained to Scott that many physical problems begin with the invasion in the body of either a poisonous substance or harmful organism. Whenever a harmful substance enters the body, the immune system police surround and engulf this foreign invader, creating what is known as an *immune complex.* A healthy body contains the enzymes necessary to eliminate immune complexes. All too often, however, junk food diets leave the body without the necessary protein building blocks to rebuild damaged cells. Poor eating habits also tend to deplete the body of antioxidants that fight cell death. And foreign substances promote the chance of allergic reaction and the buildup of immune complexes in the blood.

This chapter examines noninvasive, nonchemical means that help restore memory function by lessening the neurotoxic load of heavy metals and other toxins stored in body fat. Once this load is lessened, the immune system is enhanced, and memory cells in the brain can function better. This chapter will focus on three of these methods—NAET, niacin detoxification saunas, and fasting.

These noninvasive techniques for lowering body toxicity for the purpose of protecting brain tissue can be effective treatment options. Of course, before undertaking one of these or any other treatment method, be sure to consult with a qualified health-care provider first. *Never self-treat.* All programs should be performed under the watchful eye of a qualified doctor.

NAET ALLERGY ELIMINATION

NAET is a unique blend of both Western and Eastern healing methods that reduces and gradually eliminates allergic responses and inflammation in the body's nervous system. In the early 1980s, through a dynamic and unusual blend of kinesiology, acupressure, and acupuncture, Dr. Devi Nambudripad, DC, RN, LAc, PhD, of Buena Park, California, developed a treatment for changing the way in which a body responds to a perceived allergen. This treatment has been successful in eliminating allergies without shots, drugs, surgery, or any other invasive entry. Named after her, the treatment is called Nambudripad's Allergy Elimination Technique (NAET). Through it, thousands of patients have found allergy relief from such sources as foods, radiation, electromagnetic force fields, heavy metals, industrial chemicals, clothing fibers, soaps, and cosmetics.

As the word spread of this effective treatment, patients from all over the United States and the world began flooding Dr. Nambudripad's Buena Park clinic. When her patient load became too great, Dr. Nambudripad began training other doctors in her technique. To date, over 1,500 health-care practitioners, including medical doctors, licensed acupuncturists, chiropractors, nutritionists, herbalists, and osteopaths, have been trained to offer NAET in cities throughout the United States. Doctors in the Middle East, Western Europe, and Asia also practice NAET.

The Principle Behind NAET

NAET is based on the principle that all matter is held together by energy fields. In the human body, energy flows through nerve pathways. When the body's energy is able to flow freely through these pathways, the body is in homeostasis—a state of balance.

Dr. Nambudripad believes that any trauma—those caused by foods, chemicals, emotional events, and electric or magnetic fields—can create an energy blockage in nerve pathways. Because of this blockage, whenever the body encounters the "trauma substance," an allergic reaction results. This allergic reaction is actually a signal from your autonomic nervous system—a signal telling you to stay away from that particular substance. These blockages can put a strain on the nervous system, as well as the immune and endocrine systems. Eventually these energy blockages result in illness.

Through the unique NAET program, these blockages in the nerve pathways are broken up. Once the pathways are clear, the energy is able to flow freely, and the body is free from the allergic reaction.

While some people respond faster than others, it usually takes one treatment to clear an individual allergen. If the treatment fails, re-treatment is necessary. Generalized symptoms of poor health often require eight to twelve months of weekly treatments. Those with severe allergic responses to a number of substances may need two to three years of NAET.

The Procedure for NAET

The first step an NAET specialist takes is to discover the source and type of allergen that is causing blockage on the energy pathways. This is done through a common diagnostic tool called *muscle testing*. The patient holds a suspected allergen in his or her hand, then holds that arm out straight and taut. The specialist then begins to gently push the patient's extended arm downward toward the floor. If the patient can provide resistance to the force of the push, he or she is not allergic to the substance. If, however, the patient is unable to offer resistance, the substance is a likely allergen.

Once the allergen has been identified, the patient is asked to hold the allergen in one hand while lying on his or her stomach. Using a thumb or a special device, the specialist uses gentle pressure to stimulate energy flow in the ascending and descending nerve tracts of the spine. This pressure encourages the breaking up of energy blockages that are caused by the allergen being held in the patient's hand during the treatment.

After the pressure has been applied, the patient is muscle tested again. If the test indicates that the patient is no longer showing reactions to the allergen, he or she is treated with acupuncture needles, which seal in the treatment. Once the needles are removed (usually after twenty minutes), the patient is muscle tested a final time to be certain the treatment is successful.

For the next twenty-five hours, the patient is not permitted to taste, smell, or touch the allergen for which he or she is being treated. This is the length of time it takes for regular energy to circulate throughout all of the body's nerve centers. Any contact with the allergen during this time will cause the NAET treatment to fail. Once this energy circulation has occurred, amazingly, the patient will be cleared of the allergic response.

Many patients have reported that positive changes in the body continue to develop long after the initial energy blockage. Take forty-seven-year-old Betty, for example. Plagued with short-term memory loss and a growing inability to concentrate at work, Betty began NAET treatments for her allergic reaction to caffeine. Consuming foods or beverages with caffeine caused her thumb joints to swell up, turn red, and eventually protrude outward as well. Like many people, Betty was also unable to sleep after ingesting caffeine. Within two weeks of receiving NAET, the inflammation in her thumb joints was gone. Three months later, the joints had returned to their natural position. But the positive effects of the treatment continued. Fifteen months following NAET, Betty was able to enjoy a cup of caffeinated coffee late in the evening without it hampering her sleep.

The most exciting thing for Betty was that after thirteen months of NAET treatments, she began to retrieve her short-term memory—a plus she had not expected. Allergies affecting memory are not well understood by medical science. But with new treatments like NAET it doesn't matter, as long as memory can be safely restored and protected.

Finding a Trained NAET Practitioner

Doctors practicing NAET must also have a license or professional degree in acupuncture, chiropractic science, osteopathy, nutrition, or traditional medicine. A growing number of medical doctors in the United States are becoming NAET specialists as well. Most large cities in the United States have at least two NAET trained doctors.

Each summer, the NAET Pain Clinic and Research Foundation sponsors a professional conference where NAET doctors share their experiences with allergy elimination. The general public is invited to attend these conferences. To request a copy of the professional papers presented at these annual conferences, contact the NAET Research Foundation, 6714 Beach Boulevard, Buena Park, California, 90621; 714–523–8900. This foundation also offers a registry of NAET treatment centers throughout the United States.

A Final Note on NAET

Developed in the 1980s to curb pain and inflammatory response to allergies, the full range of treatment possibilities using NAET are not known at this time. In Israel, for example, Samuel Hendler, MD, has used NAET to treat both malignant and benign tumors. He claims that this treatment has been successful with at least thirty terminally ill cancer patients, including his father, who had prostate cancer.

The proof of NAET's effectiveness in alleviating allergies is seen in the growing number of patients who readily testify that after treatment their allergies are gone and have not returned. We believe this established ability of NAET to reduce allergic response may offer one of the best ways of cooling off cellular inflammation in the brain's memory tissue.

NIACIN DETOXIFICATION SAUNAS

The niacin detoxification sauna is another noninvasive method of restoring memory loss by lowering the levels of neurotoxic substances lodged in body fat. Some of these substances include polychlorinated biphenyls (PCBs), used in industrial coolants and lubricating agents; polybromated biphenyls (PBBs), found in fire retardants and transformers; and chlorinated chemicals, commonly used in pesticides. As 60 percent of the brain is composed of fatty tissue, lowering any buildup of fat-stored toxins can help improve memory.

The concept of a sauna—a good old-fashioned "sweat" to rid the body of toxins—goes back thousands of years. Health researcher and writer L. Ron Hubbard is believed to be the first person to use niacin (vitamin B_3) in conjunction with dry-heat saunas. During the 1960s, Hubbard's research showed that the niacin detox sauna is an effective way to dislodge and remove neurotoxic poisons that are locked in body fat.

In the early 1970s, a tragedy in Michigan helped prove the competency of these treatments. The fire retardant PBB was accidentally substituted as a dietary supplement in the feed of dairy cows and cattle, and quickly infiltrated the food chain. Contaminated meat, milk, and other foods began affecting the health of thousands of people, who started displaying a host of neurotoxic symptoms, including memory loss, headaches, inability to concentrate, and mood swings.

Seven years later, a team from the Mount Sinai School of Medicine studied the aftermath of this disaster. Tissue samples of those who had been affected showed that massive amounts of PBBs were still present. Those involved in the study were invited to undergo the Hubbard niacin detox method to eliminate the high toxin levels. After the basic sauna protocol of three weeks, PBB levels dropped by more than 20 percent. Four months after completion of the treatment, the levels had dropped by 42 percent.

A cardiologist in Florida learned of the Michigan study, and tried the same detox method on one of his patients who had been exposed to Agent Orange (dioxin). Initially, the patient's dioxin levels decreased by 29 percent. By the end of the treatment, the levels had dropped by 97 percent.

In a controlled U.S. study, electrical workers subjected to daily contact with hexachlorobenzene (HCB), PCBs, and other neurotoxic substances, underwent the Hubbard detoxification method. Researchers reported that 30 percent of the HCBs and 16 percent of the PCBs were removed as a result of the treatment.

These studies are impressive, but be aware that removal of certain toxins can be dangerous to the kidneys and liver. Individuals must be carefully monitored. It is, therefore, very important that such a detoxification program be performed under the expert guidance of a person who is qualified in supervising this treatment method.

How the Hubbard Method of Niacin Detox Works

A niacin detox sauna is based on the ability of niacin to move fat-stored toxins from the tissues into the bloodstream where it is eliminated mainly through sweat, urine, and feces.

During this treatment program, niacin (vitamin B_3) is taken to increase blood circulation throughout the body. Generally, 50 milligrams of niacin is the amount given at the onset of the program, usually just before the exercise segment of the treatment. The niacin causes what is commonly known as a "niacin flush," a temporary slight tingling or stinging sensation under the skin that is accompanied by a mild rash. Researchers believe the flush is a sign that fat-held toxins are being moved from the cells to the blood for excretion. After a few days, the niacin will no longer result in the flush, so the dosage must be increased.

Some people claim they look forward to the niacin flush because it reminds them that poisons are leaving their bodies. If this sensation makes you uncomfortable, however, minimize it by taking the niacin with food. Yogurt is a good choice. Tablet or capsule niacin is the recommended form, which has never been implicated in any serious side effects. The time-released form of niacin should not be used as it has been associated with liver problems. Niacinamide, which does not mobilize fat into the blood effectively, should be avoided as well.

In the same manner in which your car's dirty oil is replaced by clean oil during an oil change, "dirty" fat is replaced by "clean" fat in the body during niacin detox sauna treatments. In other words, fat-stored toxins are flushed from the body and replaced by clean oil that the body needs for good health. At the end of each daily treatment, the detox supervisor will supply you with your "oil change"—one to two tablespoons of high-quality, cold-pressed monounsaturated or polyunsaturated oil. The amount of oil—which is based on a number of variables, including weight gain and loss—will be determined by your supervisor.

Treatment length will depend on your toxicity levels (determined by a hair analysis), as well as the results of your physical exam. The average program runs for twenty-four consecutive days. It includes a twenty-minute workout period followed by three to five saunas—thirty minutes each—per day. There is a ten-minute cool-down period between saunas.

The Detox Sauna Experience

The following steps detail the procedure involved in the Hubbard niacin detoxification program. Once again, it is strongly recommended that this procedure be done under the guidance of one who is qualified in supervising this treatment method.

Before starting the first sauna of the day, your detox supervisor will prepare a calcium-magnesium "cocktail" by mixing 5 rounded teaspoons of calcium/magnesium powder (with an acidic base) in 2 cups of water. You will be taking this a little later.

After taking the recommended dosage of niacin, preferably with a half cup of yogurt, a twenty- to thirty-minute exercise period of running or fast walking is required to get the niacin circulating. Expect to feel the niacin flush during this time. After the exercise period, drink one cup of the calcium-magnesium mixture, and enter the sauna.

The sauna must have a controllable thermostat to keep the temperature between 140°F and 160°F. Temperatures above or below this range will be ineffective in removing toxins from body tissue. The sauna should last between twenty and thirty minutes—no longer.

After the sauna, rest comfortably and allow your body to cool down for ten minutes (no more, no less). Sit quietly and perhaps read a book. This is a critical part of the detoxification process. After the cool down, step into a quick lukewarm shower and use a clean sponge to rub your skin. This will help open the pores for more toxin excretion. Avoid the urge to take a dip in the pool or sit in a Jacuzzi. After the shower, return to the sauna for the next "sweat" session. If you feel weak after the third sauna (the minimum amount required), do not take any more that day. At the onset of this treatment program, you may need to build up gradually to the optimal five saunas. Your supervisor will help you make these decisions.

After the last sauna of the day, finish the remaining calcium-magnesium drink. End the session by taking the recommended amount of "clean" replacement oil. Taking the oil is crucial in preventing reabsorption of the toxins back into the body.

For the duration of the program, be sure to eat nutritious high-fiber meals (avoid red meat, high-fat foods, and all dairy products except yogurt), and try to get eight to ten hours of sleep each day. Whenever you feel tired or worn out, be sure to rest.

Important Considerations

Before undergoing niacin detox, it is strongly advised that you discuss your plans with your primary health-care provider. It is also important to have a complete physical examination, including a stress test and an electrocardiogram. Detox saunas can be dangerous for those with cardiovascular problems. Pregnant women and anyone with cancer or AIDS should avoid this treatment as well.

Those with a history of recreational drug use should be aware that drug flashbacks can occur during treatment.

To determine the body's heavy metal levels, a hair analysis, a twenty-four hour urine analysis, or a blood analysis are recommended. Sweating during the saunas not only eliminates fat-stored toxins, it also drains important vitamins and minerals, which can cause further memory loss. In addition, those with memory loss are typically deficient in vitamins and minerals to begin with. For these reasons, it is more important than ever to supplement with the proper nutrients—a well-rounded regimen of vitamins, minerals, antioxidants, amino acids, and enzymes—at this time. Your qualified supervisor will guide you in determining your supplement needs.

Drinking enough pure water—filtered or distilled—during these treatments is crucial. Two to three quarts during the daily series of saunas is recommended. The saunas pull a large amount of water from the body. This water is filled with sodium, potassium, calcium, and magnesium. As discussed in the previous paragraph, these minerals must be replaced. Never drink chlorinated tap water during the niacin detox or you will be defeating part of the cleansing effect. Drinking fresh, raw vegetable juice is also recommended, as are fresh-squeezed fruit juices, which help keep sugar circulating to the brain.

During the treatment, it is not uncommon to experience headaches, which are signs of dehydration and/or mineral loss. At the first sign of a headache, notify your supervisor, who will give you the proper supplements (usually salt tablets and minerals) to alleviate the discomfort. On a properly managed program, headaches and/or dizziness should not occur at all. Do not stop the saunas once you have begun.

Be sure to consume lots of fresh greens, raw and lightly steamed vegetables, and fiber-rich whole grains at mealtime. Limit your intake of meats and fats. A nutritious meal is strongly recommended before the first sauna.

Wear a comfortable bathing suit during the saunas and have a pair of rubber thongs or sandals on your feet. Do not take printed material like magazines, books, and newspapers into the sauna. The heat will activate the toxins found in the printing inks—exactly the type of neurotoxic material you are trying to remove from your body.

Finally, you should not take a niacin detox sauna alone in the event of an emergency. Most treatment centers encourage the buddy system. Having a partner who is also going through the program, either someone you know or someone appointed by the center, is a good idea. The saunas are much more enjoyable when shared with another person.

For additional information on this detoxification method, read *Clear Body, Clear Mind* by L. Ron Hubbard (Bridge Publications, 1990).

Niacin Detox Can Trigger Past Experiences

Prior psychological and/or physical experiences can be triggered during a niacin detox. As minute amounts of stored toxins pass back through tissue into the blood, original responses to these toxins can be restimulated. For instance, people who had taken LSD back in the 1970s reportedly have experienced "flashbacks" to former hallucinogenic states during detox saunas.

There was one interesting case of a forty-one-year-old woman who had had a kidney infection six months before she began her detox saunas. During the final week of her two-month treatment series, this woman experienced another kidney infection—the result of the movement of toxins from her tissues to her blood. She was put on antibiotics immediately.

This ability of toxins to restimulate past psychological and physical experiences is another reason it is important to undergo this treatment with expert supervision.

Where Are Niacin Detox Saunas Offered?

As mentioned earlier, niacin detox saunas should be performed under the expert guidance of a professional who is qualified in supervising this technique. A number of centers located throughout the United States offer this treatment. For names and addresses of some of these centers, see the Resource List, beginning on page 199.

FASTING

A carefully controlled and regulated three- to seven-day juice fast every six months is another effective method for reducing toxic buildup in the body. Pollutants in the air we breathe, as well as chemicals in the food and water we consume, all add to the body's toxic overload. Fasting is an effective and safe method of helping the body detoxify itself. Supplemented with plenty of fiber, a juice fast helps reduce body toxicity while reducing the workload of the immune system, liver, and kidneys. It helps purify and rejuvenate the blood, reducing inflammation and increasing oxygenation. As seen earlier, oxygenated blood is very important in maintaining healthy memory neurons in the brain. As an added bonus, fasting is inexpensive.

Although the basic fasting method is the water fast, it is not generally recommended. Toxins are released too quickly during an all-water fast, commonly causing reactions such as fatigue and headaches. A juice fast is preferred because of its gentler approach. Juices add essential nutrients—vitamins, minerals, enzymes—to the body. This type of fast also accustoms one to the taste of raw vegetables, encouraging the continuation of a healthy diet once the fast is over.

A fast accomplishes different things depending on its length. For instance, a three- to four-day fast is generally used to rid the body of toxins and to cleanse the blood, while a five- to seven-day fast begins the process of healing a compromised immune system. A one-day fast is sometimes a good way to start if you have never fasted before (although the hunger pangs experienced are usually strongest the first day of a fast). Fasting once or twice a year is recommended.

If you are in moderately good health and plan to fast for more than three days, be sure to do so only under the guidance of a health-care professional. Those with chronic health problems such as diabetes or hypoglycemia should not fast for even one day without their doctor's supervision. Pregnant and lactating women should never fast.

Preparing for a Fast

To prepare for the juice fast, you'll need to stock up on a few items. A good health food store with organic produce—specifically lemons and beets—will likely have everything you'll need. Unless you are planning to purchase prepared fresh lemon and beet juices for the fast, you will need a juicer. Although an electric type is recommended for speed and efficiency, a glass or plastic hand juicer can be used as well.

During this fast, you'll need about fifteen psyllium fiber capsules a day, so be sure to purchase a good-sized bottle. Fiber is necessary as it provides enough bulk to encourage peristalsis and to
absorb material for waste excretion. It also prevents weakness and
hunger. When taking fiber, large amounts of water must be consumed as well. If you have problems taking capsules, purchase
psyllium fiber in powdered form (bulk powder is less expensive
than capsules), and mix it with water. If you prepare a drink with
powdered psyllium, know that it will thicken quickly, so be sure to
drink it immediately.

The juice of fresh lemons is a great cleanser for an overworked
liver. During this fast, you will be drinking the juice of eight to sixteen lemons a day, so consider purchasing a few dozen at once to
have on hand. Try to choose those that have been organically
grown and are pesticide-free. Do not use lemon concentrate, which
lacks active bioflavonoids and does not have the proper pH level.
Though a fresh lemon starts out acidic, by the time it gets into your
digestive system, it has become alkaline.

You may want to add a little whole raw sugar to the lemon
water during the fast to help feed and energize memory tissue.
Molasses, honey, or pure maple syrup can be added as well, but do
not overdo it (you want your pancreas to rest from its insulin activities). And do not consume refined sugar of any kind or you will
defeat the fast's cleansing purpose.

As beet juice is rich in vitamin B, it is a crucial part of this fast.
If you have a juicer, plan on squeezing some fresh beet juice each
day. If you do not own a juicer, you can purchase fresh beet juice in
most health food stores. Root vegetables contain high levels of oxygen. When beets are juiced raw, memory cells reap the full benefit
of this oxygen. More important, beet juice helps move toxic excre-
tions out of the body through the digestive tract. Beet crystals,
which are added to distilled or filtered water, are also available.
Although fresh juice should always be your first choice, these crystals are an adequate substitute.

While not mandatory, a blend of nutrient-rich fresh celery, car-
rot, and parsley juice can be taken during the fast as well. This
blend is sold in most health food stores. Simply dilute eight to sixteen ounces of this juice blend in equal amounts of distilled or filtered water, and sip it throughout the day.

Be sure to have plenty of distilled or filtered water on hand.
Throughout each day of the fast, you will be consuming a mini-

mum of thirty-two ounces. Avoid tap water, which can contain traces of heavy metals, pesticides, and other toxic substances.

The Fast

Eating raw vegetables and fruits is recommended for the two days prior to starting the fast. It will make the fast less of a shock to the body.

On the first day of the fast, in the early morning, mix the juice of six to eight fresh lemons with thirty-two ounces of distilled water. Immediately drink sixteen ounces of this lemon water along with six psyllium fiber capsules. Mid-morning, drink the rest of the lemon water and take another six psyllium capsules.

In the early afternoon, squeeze another six to eight lemons and mix the juice with another thirty-two ounces of water. Drink half of this mixture for lunch and the other half during the afternoon. It is best to drink this all at once. You can drink the beet juice anytime during the day. (Drink two ounces on the first day, four ounces on the second, and six ounces on the third and any remaining days.) By the second day of the fast, many people begin to experience a cooling sensation in their bodies along with an abundance of energy. Some report a sudden, "clarity of thinking."

The first few day on the fast is likely to be the most difficult because you'll probably be feeling strong hunger pangs. If this happens, take an additional two or three psyllium capsules and drink more lemon water. The fasting will get easier each day. You will know it's time to stop the fast if you begin to feel fatigued after having felt energetic, experience unusual hunger, or notice you are losing weight. For most people, a three to five day fast will bring excellent detox results.

Ending the Fast

Breaking a fast should be given the same attention that was given to the fast itself. If you break the fast with a heavy meal, you are likely to experience stomach cramps. Begin gradually by eating small, simple meals consisting of raw or lightly steamed vegetables and fresh fruits. Chew the food well, keep food combinations simple, and do not overeat. Reduce your intake of psyllium by 50 percent, but continue drinking plenty of filtered water.

For the next few days, depending on how well your body is

adjusting to the transition, you can add some whole grains and legumes to your diet. Be sure to keep the meals simple and healthy. Eventually begin a gradual reintroduction of carbohydrates like pasta, bread, and potatoes. After the fast, consume only moderate amounts of fat-laden dairy products, and do not eat more than three ounces of red meat or poultry in a day. Continue taking two to three fiber capsules daily.

CONCLUSION

NAET treatments, Hubbard niacin detox saunas, and juice fasts, as well as the chelation and oxygen healing therapies discussed in Chapter 8, are cutting-edge strategies you can use to reduce your body's toxic load. Lowered toxicity levels result in an enhanced immune system and memory cells that can function better.

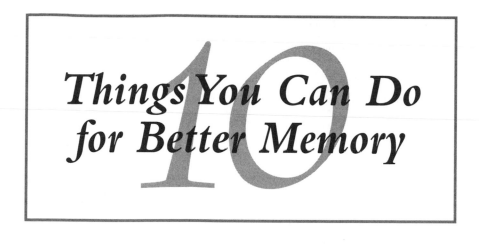

Things You Can Do for Better Memory

*"Very little is needed to make a happy life.
It is all within yourself, in your way of thinking."*

—Marcus Aurelius

Some memory boosters limit the neurotoxic effects of flavor enhancers, heavy metals, and pesticides. Others work to prevent oxygen starvation and maintain energy levels in memory cells. Still others protect neuronal membranes, while some enhance neurotransmitter production. All of the suggested techniques—presented in detail throughout the book—have been summarized below for quick reference. Remember, no matter what your age, no matter how much brain loss you have experienced at this time, at least some of the following suggestions will enable you to help support and strengthen your existing neurons.

1. *Avoid processed foods, which typically contain chemical food additives, including preservatives, color, and flavor enhancers.*

2. *Whenever possible, choose organically grown produce, as well as meat and poultry from organically raised free-range animals.*

3. *Eat plenty of enzyme-rich raw foods.*

4. *Limit dietary fat intake to 20 percent of the total calories consumed each day.*

5. *Limit intake of processed sugar.*

6. *Limit caffeine intake.*

7. *Avoid heavy alcohol consumption.*

8. *Avoid recreational drugs.*

9. *Drink only clean filtered water, free of heavy metals, pesticides, or solvents.*

10. *Shower with clean filtered water to avoid neurotoxin absorption through the skin.*

11. *Be aware of the benefits of omega-3 fatty acids for good memory. Take 1 to 2 tablespoons of a reliable source of these essential oils daily. To assist the good work of omega-3 oils, decrease consumption of red meat, eggs, and dairy products.*

12. *When taking fish oil supplements as a rich source of beneficial omega-3 fatty acids, be sure the oil comes from fish caught in deep, cold ocean waters only. Fish caught in inland waters may contain neurotoxic substances. Be sure the product label carries a third-party safety verification.*

13. *Limit the use of antibiotics and other prescription drugs. When antibiotics are necessary, however, be sure to accompany them with L. acidophilus, B. bifidus, L. bulgaricus, and other friendly bacteria, which will help build up their beneficial colonies in the gastrointestinal tract.*

14. *Avoid using toxic insecticides inside or outside your home.*

15. *Keep a safe distance from electrical appliances, which emit possible harmful electromagnetic rays. This includes the little black boxes attached to small electrical gadgets such as desktop calculators and telephone answering machines.*

16. *Avoid stressful situations and practice calming techniques to encourage relaxation. Stop multi-tasking behavior.*

17. *Once a year after age forty, consider a supervised detoxification sauna program to eliminate any fat-stored toxins from your system.*

18. *Use an air filter to purify the air in your home, car, and workplace.*

19. *Get at least eight hours of continuous sleep in complete darkness each night.*

20. *At least three times a week, perform some cardiovascular exercise—*

swimming, walking, jogging, or riding a bicycle for instance—for at least twenty minutes.

21. *If you suffer with allergies, consider NAET treatment for allergy elimination (see Chapter 9).*

22. *Discuss taking high-quality memory-enhancing supplements with your health-care provider.*

23. *Replace mercury amalgam dental fillings to avoid heavy metal toxicity.*

24. *Do not use aluminum cookware or utensils.*

25. *Do not use baking powder that contains aluminum when making baked goods. Instead, use baking powder made of calcium acid phosphate, cornstarch, and bicarbonate of soda. Avoid commercial baked goods made with baking powder that contains aluminum. Check product labels for "aluminum-free" baking powder in the in-gredient list.*

26. *Do not use laxatives or deodorants that contain aluminum.*

27. *Use only cosmetics that are free of aluminum lakes.*

28. *Avoid nail polish and polish removers that contain formaldehyde or toluene.*

29. *Avoid using hair dye or bleach.*

30. *Consider chelation therapy for reducing toxic heavy metal buildup in your system.*

31. *Do not buy furniture made with particle board, which is held to-gether with neurotoxic glues and solvents.*

32. *Limit exposure to petrochemicals, including those used in carpeting and other floor coverings, paints and paint removers, wallpaper, waxes, and furniture polish.*

Lifelong memory is like a concerto for which you want a rous-ing good ending. No matter what your age, small, but significant changes in your daily routine will help support your memory function. When physical, nutritional, and mental stresses are lifted from memory pathways, the immune system can be strengthened, reducing inflammation in memory tissue. Keeping nutrient levels high will help maintain adequate glucose levels and increase energy conversion in memory nerve cells. Such simple, yet decisive steps, can help you reduce free radical damage and lower neurotoxic influences. As a result, you will more likely be able to remember the important details of life.

Remember, although some memory loss is normal as you age, severe memory loss is not necessarily inevitable. What's important is that you have the power to help restore lost memory neurons and strengthen existing ones. Make a sincere effort to follow the suggestions outlined above (and detailed in the earlier chapters of this book) to help maximize your precious memory. You owe it to yourself.

Glossary

Acetylcholine. Considered the brain's most important neurotransmitter for memory and thinking, acetylcholine is crucial for message transmission.

Alzheimer's disease. A degenerative disorder characterized by physiological changes in the brain that cause impaired memory and thought processes.

Amygdala. The emotional processing center of the limbic system.

Arteriosclerosis. A circulatory disorder characterized by a thickening and stiffening of the walls of arteries, which impedes circulation.

Atherosclerosis. The most common type of arteriosclerosis, caused by the accumulation of fatty deposit buildup on artery walls.

Autonomic nervous system. The part of the central nervous system that controls unconscious bodily functions, such as breathing and heartbeat.

Axon. The part of a memory neuron that carries information to another memory neuron.

Basal ganglia (striatum). Located deep in the cerebrum, the basal ganglia plays a significant part in unconscious, automatic body movements.

Brain stem. The part of the brain that connects the base of the cerebrum to the spinal cord. It controls body functions like balance, breathing, sensory and motor nerves, and heart rate.

Cerebrovascular accident (CVA). More commonly known as a stroke, a CVA is caused by lack of blood flow and insufficient oxygen to the brain, resulting in death of brain tissue. High blood pressure and atherosclerosis are the two most common causes.

Cerebellum. The part of the brain that coordinates body movements.

Cerebrum. The largest part of the brain, the cerebrum houses most of the capabilities for thinking and intelligence. It is divided into two halves—the right half governs aspects of creativity and non-verbal communication, while the left half is responsible for logical thinking as well as written and verbal expression.

Corpus callosum. The part of the brain that connects the right and left hemispheres of the cerebrum.

Dendrite. The part of a memory neuron that receives information from an axon.

Explicit memory. Conscious memory.

Free radical. An unpaired electron seeking a stable bond with another electron. Groups of such radicals or electrons attack healthy tissue, leaving behind more unpaired electrons.

Frontal lobe. The area of the cerebrum that is considered the primary seat of memory. The frontal lobe governs abstract thinking and speech.

Glia cells. Caretakers of neurons.

Hemorrhagic stroke. The type of stroke in which a blood vessel bursts, preventing normal blood flow to the brain and causing blood leakage.

Hippocampus. The area of the limbic system where short-term memory is stored until a decision is made whether or not to ship that memory to long-term storage in the cerebral cortex. The hippocampus focuses on conscious memory of "unemotional" data—events, places, and facts.

Hypertension. High blood pressure.

Hypothalamus. A portion of the brain that regulates immune function, the autonomic nervous system, mood and motivational states, and many aspects of metabolism, such as hunger and body temperature. It is not protected by the blood-brain barrier.

Immune complex. Cellular "garbage" that is created when the immune system "police" surround and engulf foreign invaders. A healthy body contains the enzymes necessary to eliminate immune complexes.

Implicit memory. Unconscious memory.

Ischemic stroke. The type of stoke in which blood flow to the brain is stopped due to a blocked blood vessel. This blockage is generally caused either by atherosclerosis or a blood clot.

Limbic system. A cluster of neurons deep inside the brain in which emotional reactions to stimuli take place. It is made up of the hippocampus, the amygdala, the hypothalamus, the thalamus, and the pituitary. Each of these specialized neuron clusters has a distinct function that supports cognition and memory.

Memory. The storage of all learning. The main types include working memory, which lasts a few seconds; short-term memory, which is retained from a few hours to several days, and long-term memory, which gets stored away forever.

Metabolism. The physical and chemical processes necessary to sustain life, including the production of cellular energy.

Mitochondria. The part of a cell in which oxygen and blood sugar are converted into cellular energy.

Myelin sheath. In much the same way that insulation surrounds an electrical wire, the myelin sheath coats the axons of a neuron.

Neuron. A memory cell that receives, processes, saves, and sends messages. It is composed of a body, an axon, and dendrites.

Neurotransmitters. The chemical carriers that enable memory information to cross over synapses (spaces) between neurons. Without these important biochemical carriers, memory would not be possible.

Nootropics. An ancient Greek term that means "acting on the mind." Nootropics is a modern term for "smart" drugs, substances believed to improve existing memory or to prevent memory loss.

Occipital lobe. The area of the cerebrum that regulates sight.

Parasympathetic nervous system. The part of the autonomic nervous system that regulates the ongoing processes of temperature regulation, resting, and digestion.

Parietal lobes. The area of the cerebrum that integrates all sensory information. It is where the capability for analytical reasoning and logical deduction are found.

Parkinson's disease. A degenerative disease that affects the nervous system, Parkinson's disease is associated with a lack of the neurotransmitter dopamine. It is characterized by uncontrollable tremors, muscle stiffness, and fatigue. Thirty-two percent of those with this disease develop dementia.

Pituitary. A gland located at the base of the brain that secretes hormones. Pituitary hormones regulate growth and metabolism.

Plasticity. The ability of existing neurons to increase their storage capacity through new learning experiences.

Positron emission transmission (PET) scan. Sometimes referred to as "real time" images, PET scans allow researchers to track and record which memory centers get stimulated in live, working brain tissue during memory processing.

Sphygmomanometer. A device that measures blood pressure.

Stroke. *See* Cerebrovascular accident.

Synapse. The gap or space between neurons.

Temporal lobes. The part of the cerebrum that coordinates the awareness and interpretation of sounds and language. Musical skills like singing, playing an instrument, and composing are centered here. Temporal lobes allow people to recognize other people and objects, process and retrieve long-term memories, and initiate communication or action.

Thalamus. A part of the brain that organizes sensory materials.

Transient ischemic attack (TIA). A brief, temporary disruption in brain function caused by insufficient blood flow. It is sometimes referred to as a minor stroke. Generally the result of a temporary blockage in one of the small blood vessels leading to the brain, a transient ischemic attack is more likely to occur in those with high blood pressure, atherosclerosis, or heart disease.

Traumatic brain injury. A closed-head or open-head injury to the brain. In an open-head injury, the skull is penetrated, such as from a gunshot wound. In a closed-head injury, the skull is not penetrated, but the brain is injured from an external force, such as a sudden jolt that causes the brain to move inside the skull.

Resource List

Homeopathic Pharmacies

The following pharmacies carry pharmaceutical-quality supplements. All provide mail order service.

Abrams Royal Pharmacy
8220 Abrams Road
Dallas, TX 75231
Phone: 214–349–8000
    800–458–0804
Fax: 214–341–7966

College Pharmacy
3505 Austin Bluff Parkway,
   Suite 101
Colorado Springs, CO 80918
Phone: 719–262–0022
    800–888–9358
Fax: 719–262–0035
    800–556–5893
Email: collegep@RMI.net
www.collegepharmacy.com

Hickey Chemists
888 Second Avenue
New York, NY 10017

Phone: 212–223–6333
    800–724–5566
Fax: 212–980–1533
www.JerryHickey.com

Santa Monica Homeopathic
   Pharmacy
629 Broadway
Santa Monica, CA 90401
Phone: 310–395–1131
Fax: 310–595–7861
Email:
   smhomeopathic@hotmail.com

Willner Chemists
100 Park Avenue
New York, NY 10017
Phone: 212–682–2817
    800–633–1106
Fax: 212–682–6192
Email:
   Dongold@mindspring.com

International Sources of "Smart" Drugs

The following reputable companies carry a number of "smart" drugs from sources outside the United States.

International Antiaging
   Systems (IAS)
PO Box 337J
Channel Islands GYI
Great Britain
Phone: 011–44–541–514144
Fax: 011–44–541–514145
Email:
  ias(j)@antiaging-systems.com
www.antiaging-systems.com

Quality Health, Inc.
401 Langham House
29–30 Margaret Street
London, W1N 7LB England
Fax: 011–44–171–580–2043
Email: Sales@qhi.co.uk
www.qhi.co.uk

Niacin Detoxification Sauna Centers

Health Med
5501 Power In Road, Suite 140
Sacramento, CA 95820
Phone: 916–387–6929

Purification Program
Scientology Information
   Center
6331 Hollywood Boulevard,
   Suite 1305
Los Angeles, CA 90028
Phone: 800–367–8788

This organization offers programs throughout the country. Call for locations of the treatment centers nearest you. You do not have to be a member of the Church of Scientology to utilize this program.

Notes

Chapter 1 How Memory Works

Ackerman, S. *Discovering the Brain*. Washington, DC: The National Academy Press, 1992.

Aggleton, J., editor. *The Amygdala*. New York: Wiley-Liss, 1992.

Blaylock, R. *Excitotoxins: The Taste That Kills*. Santa Fe, New Mexico: Health Press, p. 297, 1997.

Conn, M., editor. *Neuroscience in Medicine*. Philadelphia: J. B. Lippincott Company, 1995.

Elman, J. "Learning and development in neural networks: the importance of starting small." *Cognition*, 48(1): 71–99, 1993.

Kalaria, R. "Serum amyloid P in Alzheimer's disease: Implications for dysfunction of the blood brain barrier." *Annals New York Academy of Science*, 640: 145–148, 1991.

Kandel, E. *Essentials of Neural Science and Behavior*. Stamford, CT: Appellation & Lane, 1995.

Kolata, G. "Studies find brain grows new cells." *The New York Times*, B9, B12, March 17, 1998.

Lewis, D. "Intracellular regulation of ion channels in cell membranes." *Mayo Clinic Proceedings*, 65: 1127–1143, 1990.

Merck Manual of Medical Information, The. Whitehouse Station, NJ: Merck Research Laboratories, 1997.

Mooradian, A. "The effect of aging on the blood-brain barrier. A review." *Neurobiological Aging,* 9: 31–39, 1988.

Parent, A. *Carpenter's Human Neuroanatomy,* 9th edition. Baltimore: Williams & Wilkins, p. 1011, 1996.

Siegal, G., editor. *Basic Neurochemistry.* New York: Raven Press, 1989.

Winocur, G. "A neuropsychological analysis of memory loss with age." *Neurobiology of Aging,* 9(5–6): 487–94, 1988.

Chapter 2 Why Memory Fails

Anderson, A. "Neurotoxic follies." *Psychology Today,* 30–42, July 1982.

Avdulov, N. "Amyloid beta-peptides increase annular and bulk fluidity and induce lipid peroxidation in brain synaptic plasma membranes." *Journal of Neurochemistry,* 68(5): 2086–2091, 1997.

Baxter, M. "Intact spatial learning following lesions of basal forebrain cholinergic neurons." *Neuroreport,* 7(8): 1417–20, 1996.

Bechara, A. "Failure to respond autonomically to anticipated future outcomes following damage to prefrontal cortex." *Cerebral Cortex,* 6(2): 215–225, 1996.

Grady, C. "Age-related reductions in human recognition memory due to impaired encoding." *Science,* 269(5221): 218–221, 1995.

Halliwell, B. "Antioxidants in human health and disease." *Annual Review of Nutrition,* 16: 33–50, 1996.

Harik, S. "Altered glucose metabolism in microvessels from patients with Alzheimer's disease." *Annals of Neurobiology,* 26: 91–94, 1991.

Hershey, L. "Dementia associated with stroke." *Stroke,* 21: 9–11, 1990.

Laakso, M. "MRI of amygdala fails to diagnose early Alzheimer's disease." *Neuroreport,* 6(17): 2414–2418, 1995.

Lyras, L. "An assessment of oxidative damage to proteins, lipids, and DNA in brain from patients with Alzheimer's disease." *Journal of Neurochemistry,* 68(5): 2061–2169, 1997.

Mackay, S. "Regional gray and white matter metabolite differences in subjects with AD, with subcortical ischemic vascular dementia, and elderly controls with 1H magnetic resonance spectroscopic imaging." *Archives of Neurology,* 53(2): 167–174, 1996.

McGeer, P. "The inflammatory response system of the brain: Implications for therapy of Alzheimer and other neurodegenerative diseases." *Brain Research Reviews,* 21: 195–218, 1995.

New Chemicals Program. United States Environmental Protection Agency, Office of Pollution Prevention and Toxics, EPA–734–F–95–001, May 13, 1995.

Rapp. P. "Preserved neuron number in the hippocampus of aged rats with spatial learning deficits." *Proceedings of the National Academy of Sciences of the United States of America,* 93(18): 9926–9930, 1996.

Rugg, M. "Differential activation of the prefrontal cortex in successful and unsuccessful memory retrieval." *Brain,* 119(6): 2073–2083, 1996.

Sayre, L. "4-Hydroxynonenal-derived advanced lipid peroxidation end products are increased in Alzheimer's disease." *Journal of Neurochemistry,* 6(5): 2092–2097, 1997.

Scheibel, A. "Alzheimer's disease as a capillary dementia." *Annals of Medicine,* 21: 103–107, 1989.

Singer, R. *Neurotoxicity Guidebook.* New York: Van Nostrand Reinhold, 1990.

Small, G. "Predictors of cognitive change in middle-aged and older adults with memory loss." *American Journal of Psychiatry,* 152(12): 1757–1764, 1995.

Small, G. "Age-associated memory loss: initial neuropsychological and cerebral metabolic findings of a longitudinal study." *International Psychogeriatrics,* 6(1): 23–44, 1994.

Wallin, A. "Blood-brain barrier function in vascular dementia." *ACTA, Neurological Scandinavia,* 81: 318–322, 1990.

Chapter 3 Conventional Causes of Memory Failure

Arendt, T. "Impairment in memory function and neurodegenerative changes in the cholinergic basal forebrain system induced by chronic intake of ethanol." *Journal of Neural Transmission,* Supplementum 44: 173–187, 1994.

Chui, H. "Extrapyramidal signs and psychiatric symptoms predict faster cognitive decline in Alzheimer's disease." *Archives of Neurology*, 51(7): 676–681, 1994.

Demitrack, M. "Relation of dissociative phenomena to levels of cerebrospinal fluid monoamine metabolites and beta-endorphin in patients with eating disorders: A pilot study." *Psychiatry Research*, 49(1): 1–10, 1993.

Oscar-Berman, M. "Association learning and recognition memory in alcoholic Korsakoff patients." *Neuropsychology*, 2: 282–289, 1997.

Robinson, T. "Effects of cortical serotonin depletion induced by 3,4-methylenedioxymethamphetamine (MDMA) on behavior, before and after additional cholinergic blockade." *Neuropsychopharmacology*, 8(1): 77–85, 1993.

Vernon, M. *Reversing Memory Loss*. Boston: Houghton Mifflin Company, 1992.

Vorhees, C. "Methamphetamine exposure during early postnatal development in rats." *Psychopharmacology*, 114(3): 392–401, 1994.

Chapter 4 Unsuspected Causes of Memory Failure

Cosmetics and Other Body Image Enhancements

Calkin, R. *Perfumery*. New York: John Wiley and Sons, Inc., 181–186, 1994.

Dadd, D. *Nontoxic, Natural, and Earthwise*. New York: St. Martin's Press, 1990.

Fincher, C. *Healthy Living in a Toxic World*. Colorado Springs, CO: Pinon Press, 1996.

Fisher, A. "Adverse nail reactions and paresthesia from 'photobonded acrylate sculptured nails.'" *Cutis*, 45: 293–94, 1990.

National Research Council. *Toxicity Testing, Strategies to Determine Needs and Priorities*. Washington, DC: National Academy Press, 1984.

Marks, J. *Contact and Occupational Dermatology*. St. Louis, MO: Mosby Year Book, 1992.

Murray, J. "Aluminum neurotoxicity: a re-evaluation." *Clinical Neuropharmacology*, 14: 179–185, 1991.

Novelli, J. "Glutamate becomes neurotoxic via the N-methyl-D-aspartate receptor when intracellular energy levels are reduced." *Brain Research*, 451: 205–212, 1988.

Steinman, D. *The Safe Shopper's Bible*. New York: Macmillian Publishing, 1995.

Stewart, L. "Patch testing to cosmetics and topical drugs." *American Journal of Contact Dermatitis*, 7: 53–55, 1996.

Wallace, L. "VOCs and the environment and public health exposure." H. J. Bloeman and J. Burn, editors, *Chemistry and Analysis of Volatile Organic Compounds in the Environment*. Glasgow, Scotland: Blackie Academic and Professional, 1–24, 1993.

Cleansers & Soaps

Consumer Product Safety Commission. "1990 Product Summary Report: National Electronic Injury Surveillance System." Washington, DC: National Injury Information Clearinghouse, 1990.

Fincher, C. *Healthy Living in a Toxic World*. Colorado Springs, CO: Pinon Press, 1996.

Marks, J. *Contact and Occupational Dermatology*. St. Louis, MO: Mosby Year Book, 1992.

Singer, R. *Neurotoxicity Guidebook*. New York: Van Nostrand Reinhold, 1990.

Steinman, D. *The Safe Shopper's Bible*. New York: MacMillan Publishing, 1995.

Construction Materials

Ashford, N. *Chemical Exposures*. New York: Van Nostrand Reinhold, 1991.

Randolph, T. *An Alternative Approach to Allergies*. New York: Harper & Row, 1989.

Dadd, D. *Nontoxic, Natural, and Earthwise*. New York: St. Martin's Press, 1990.

Singer, R. *Neurotoxicity Guidebook*. New York: Van Nostrand Reinhold, 1990.

Wallace, L. "VOCs and the Environment and Public Health Exposure." H.J. Bloemen and J. Burn, editors, *Chemistry and Analysis of Volatile Organic Compounds in the Environment.* Glasgow, Scotland: Blackie Academic and Professional, 1–24, 1993.

Dental Amalgams

Bellinger, D. "Longitudinal analyses of prenatal and postnatal lead exposure and early cognitive development." *New England Journal of Medicine,* 316: 1037–1043, 1987.

Casdorph, H., and M. Walker. *Toxic Metal Syndrome.* Garden City Park, NY: Avery Publishing Group, 1995.

Lussi, A. "The amalgam problems: Recommendations on patient assessment and counseling." *Schwizerische Medizinische Wochenschrift,* 127(10): 398–405, 1997.

Malt, U. "Physical and mental problems attributed to dental amalgam fillings: A descriptive study of 99 self-referred patients compared to 272 controls." *Psychosomatic Medicine,* 59(1): 32–41, 1997.

Moon, C. "Main and interaction effects of metallic pollutants on cognitive functioning." *Journal of Learning Disabilities,* 18(4): 217–221, 1985.

Oskarsson, A. "Total and inorganic mercury in breast milk and blood in relation to fish consumption and amalgam fillings in lactating women." *Archives of Environmental Health,* 51(3): 234–241, 1996.

Ratcliffe, H. "Human exposure to mercury: A critical assessment of the evidence of adverse health effects." *Journal of Toxicology and Environmental Health,* 49(3): 221–270, 1996.

Rowland, A. "The effect of occupational exposure to mercury vapor on the fertility of female dental assistants." *Occupational and Environmental Medicine,* 51(1): 28–34, 1994.

Sehnert, K. "Is mercury toxicity an autoimmune disorder?" *Townsend Letter for Doctors & Patients,* 134–137, October, 1995.

Sullivan, K. "The evidence linking silver-mercury fillings to Alzheimer's disease: a literature review." *Townsend Letter for Doctors & Patients,* August/September, 1997.

Takeuchi, T. "Pathology of Minamata disease." *Acta Pathology of Japan,* 32 (supplement 1): 73–99, 1982.

Electromagnetic Fields

Becker, R. *Cross Currents: The Perils of Electropollution, The Promise of Electromedicine.* New York: Jeremy P. Tarcher, 1990.

Feychting, M. "Dementia and occupational exposure to magnetic fields." *Scandinavian Journal of Work, Environment and Health,* 1998.

Lai, H. "Effects of a 60-Hz magnetic field on central cholinergic systems of the rat." *Bioelectromagnetics,* 14: 5–15, 1993.

Lai, H. "Acute exposure to a 60-Hz magnetic field affects rats' performance in the water maze performance." *Bioelectromagnetics,* 19: 117–122, 1998.

Lai, H. "Acute exposure to a 60-Hz magnetic field increases DNA single-strand breaks in rat brain cells." *Bioelectromagnetics,* 18: 156–165, 1997.

Lai, H. "Melatonin and a spin-trap compound blocked radio frequency radiation-induced DNA single and double strand breaks in rat brain cells." *Journal of Pineal Research,* 22: 151–162, 1997.

Levenstein, M.K. *Everyday Cancer Risks and How to Avoid Them.* Garden City Park, NY: Avery Publishing Group, 1992.

Levitt, B. *Electromagnetic Fields: A Consumer's Guide to the Issues and How to Protect Ourselves,* New York: Harcourt Brace & Company, 1995.

McEntee, W. "Glutamate: Its role in learning, memory, and the aging brain." *Psychopharmacology,* 111(4): 391–401, 1993.

McMahan, S. "Depressive symptomatology in women and residential proximity to high-voltage transmission lines." *American Journal of Epidemiology,* 139: 58–63, 1994.

Poole, C. "Depressive symptoms and headaches in relation to proximity to an alternating-current transmission line right-of-way." *American Journal of Epidemiology,* 137: 318–330, 1993.

Reiter, R. "Alterations of the circadian melatonin rhythm by the electromagnetic spectrum: a study in environmental toxicology." *Regulatory Toxicology and Pharmacology,* 15: 226–244, 1992.

Sobel, E. "Electromagnetic field exposure may cause increased production of amyloid beta and eventually lead to Alzheimer's disease." *Neurology,* 47: 1594–1600, 1996.

Excitotoxins

Blaylock, R. *Excitotoxins: The Taste That Kills.* Santa Fe, NM: Health Press, 1997.

Didier, M. "Chronic glutamate toxicity casues DNA damage." *Neurology,* 44: A236, 1994.

Siegel, G., editor. *Basic Neurochemistry.* New York: Raven Press, 1989.

Siesjo, B. "Calcium, excitotoxins, and neuronal death in the brain." *Annals of the New York Academy of Sciences,* 568: 234–251, 1989.

Schwartz, G. *In Bad Taste: The MSG Syndrome.* Sante Fe, NM: Health Press, 1988.

Weiss, J. "Differential vulnerability to excitatory amino acid-induced toxicity and selective neuronal loss in neurodegenerative disease." *Canadian Journal of Neurological Science,* 18: 394–397, 1991.

Filtration: Air and Water

Levenstein, Mary Kerney. *Everyday Cancer Risks and How to Avoid Them.* Garden City Park, NY: Avery Publishing Group, 1992.

Parasites

Abu-Shakra, M. "Parasitic infectional autoimmunity." *Autoimmunity,* 9(4): 337–344, 1991.

Crissinger, K. "Pathophysiology of gastrointestinal mucosal permeability." *Journal of Internal Medicine,* 228(1): 145–154, 1990.

Galland, L. "Intestinal protozoan infection is a common unsuspected cause of chronic illness." *Journal of Advanced Medicine,* 2: 539–552, 1989.

Jenkins, A. "Do non-steroidal anti-inflammatory drugs increase colonic permeability?" *Gut,* 32: 66–69, 1991.

Otamiri, T. "Ginkgo biloba extract prevents mucosal damage associated with small-intestinal ischaemia." *Scandinavian Journal of Gastroenterology,* 24: 666–670, 1989.

Pesticides

Albertson, T. "The effect of lindane and long-term potentiation (LTP) on pyramidal cell excitability in the rat hippocampal slice." *Neuro Toxicology*, 18(2): 469–478, 1997.

Dadd, D. *Nontoxic, Natural, and Earthwise.* New York: St. Martin's Press, 1990.

Environmental Protection Agency. "Suspended, canceled, and restricted pesticides." Washington, DC: Government Printing Office, February 1990.

"Export of pesticides is not adequately monitored by EPA." General Accounting Office, Washington, DC: GAO/RCED 89–126, 1989.

Fincher, C. *Healthy Living in a Toxic World.* Colorado Springs, CO: Pinon Press, 1996.

Golan, R. *Optimal Wellness,* New York: Ballantine Books, 1995.

Hallenbeck, W. *Pesticides and Human Health.* New York: Springer-Verlag, 1985.

Hayes, W. *Pesticides Studied In Man.* Baltimore, MD: Williams and Wilkins, 1982.

Jacobson, J. "Evidence for PCBs as neurodevelopmental toxicants in humans." *Neuro Toxicology,* 18(2): 415–425, 1997.

Jeyaratnam, J. "Acute pesticide poisoning: a major global health problem." *World Health Statistics Quarterly,* 43(3): 139–144, 1990.

Klein-Schwartz, W. "Agricultural and horticultural chemical poisoning: mortality and morbidity in the United States." *Annals of Emergency Medicine,* 29(2): 232–8, 1997.

Lifton, B. *Bug Busters.* Garden City Park, NY: Avery Publishing Group, 1991.

McConnachie, P. "Immune alterations in humans exposed to the termiticide technical chlordane." *Archives of Environmental Health,* 27: 296–297, 1992.

Meister, T., editor. *Farm Chemicals Handbook,* Willoughby, Ohio: Meister Publishing Company, 1990.

Misra, U. "A study of cognitive functions in methyl-iso-cyanate victims one year after Bhopal accident." *Neuro Toxicology,* 18(2): 381–386, 1997.

Singer, R. *Neurotoxicity Guidebook.* New York: Van Nostrand Reinhold, 1990.

Steinman, D. *Living Healthy in a Toxic World.* New York: The Berkley Publishing Group, 1996.

Wong, P. "Ortho-substituted 2,2',3,5',6-Pentachlorobiphenyl (PCB 95) alters rat hippocampal ryanodine receptors and neuroplasticity in vitro: evidence for altered hippocampal functon." *Neuro Toxicology,* 18(2): 443–456, 1997.

Chapter 5 Assessing Your Memory Loss

Crook, Thomas. Interview, March 15, 1998.

Reisberg, B. *Alzheimer's Disease: The Standard Reference.* New York: Free Press, 1983.

Reisberg, B. "Dementia staging in chronic care populations." *Alzheimer's Disease and Associated Disorders,* vol 8(1): S188–205, 1994.

Chapter 6 "Smart" Nutrients

"Alzheimer's alchemy." *Science News,* 141: 152–153, March 7, 1992.

Balch, James F., and Phyllis A. Balch. *Prescription for Nutritional Healing,* 2nd edition. Garden City Park, NY: Avery Publishing Group, 1997.

Barbiroli, B. "Lipoic (thiotic) acid increases brain energy availability and skeletal muscle performance as shown by *in vivo* 31P-MRS in a patient with mitochondria cytopathy." *Journal of Neurology,* 242 (7): 472–477, 1995.

Benton, D. "The impact of selenium supplementation on mood." *Biological Psychiatry,* 29: 1092–1098, 1991.

Blaylock, R. *Excitotoxins: The Taste That Kills.* Santa Fe, NM: Health Press, 1997.

Bonavita, E. "Study of the efficacy and tolerability of L-acetylcarnitine therapy in the senile brain." *International Journal of Clinical Pharmacology Therapy and Toxicology,* 24: 511–516, 1986.

Borgstrom, L. "Pharmacokinetics of N-acetylcysteine in man." *European Journal of Clinical Pharmacology*, 31: 271–272, 1986.

Butterworth, R. "Effects of thiamine deficiency on brain metabolism: Implications for the pathogenesis of Wernicke-Korsakoff syndrome." *Alcohol Alcoholism*, 24: 271–279, 1989.

Calvani, M. "Action of acetyl-l-carnitine in neurodegeneration and Alzheimer's disease." *Annals of the New York Academy of Science*, 663: 483–486, 1992.

Cantz, D. "Lecithin and choline in human health and disease." *Nutrition Reviews*, 52(10): 327–339, 1994.

Carney, M. "Vitamin deficiency and mental symptoms." *British Journal of Psychiatry*, 156: 878–882, 1990.

Chernoff, R. "Nutrition and aging," in Shils, M. *Modern Nutrition in Health and Disease*. Philadelphia: Lea & Febinger, 1988.

Cichoke, Anthony J. *The Complete Book of Enzyme Therapy*. Garden City Park, NY: Avery Publishing Group, 1999.

Davis, S. "Acetyl-L-carnitine: behavioral, electrophysiological, and neurochemical effects." *Neurobiology of Aging*, 14(1): 107–115, 1993.

Frizel, D. "Plasma calcium and magnesium in depression." *British Journal of Psychiatry*, 115: 1375–1377, 1969.

Fulder, Stephen. *The Ginseng Book*. Garden City Park, NY: Avery Publishing Group, 1996.

Ghadirian, A. "Folic acid deficiency and depression." *Psychosomatics*, 21(11): 926–929, 1980.

Glick, J. "Dementia: the role of magnesium deficiency and an hypothesis concerning the pathogenesis of Alzheimer's disease." *Medical Hypothesis*, 31: 211–225, 1991.

Golan, R. *Optimal Wellness*. New York: Ballantine Books, p. 533, 1995.

Halliwell, B. "Antioxidants in human health and disease." *Annual Review of Nutrition*, 16: 33–50, 1996.

Harbige, L. "Nutrition and immunity with emphasis on infection and autoimmune disease." *Nutrition and Health*, 10(4): 285–312, 1996.

Huxtable, R. "The pharmacology of extinction." *Journal of Ethnopharmacology*, 37(1): 1–11, 1992.

Jahnke, A. "Into the mouths of babes." *Psychology Today*, 26: 8, 1993.

Kleijnen, J. "Ginkgo biloba for cerebral insufficiency." *British Journal of Clinical Pharmacology*, 34: 352–358, 1992.

Langley, W. "Central nervous system magnesium deficiency." *Archives of International Medicine*, 151: 593–596, 1991.

Leaf, A. "Cardiovascular effects of omega-3 fatty acids." *New England Journal of Medicine*, 318: 549–557.

Mindell, E. *Vitamin Bible*. New York: Warner Books, p. 346, 1991.

Murray, M. *Encyclopedia of Nutritional Supplements*. Rocklin, CA: Prima Publishing, 1996.

Nagamatsu, M. "Lipoic acid improves nerve blood flow, reduces oxidative stress, and improves distal nerve conduction in experimental diabetic neuropathy." *Diabetes Care*, 18: 1160–1167, 1995.

Nasr, S. "Correction of vitamin E deficiency with fat-soluble versus water-miscible preparations of vitamin E in patients with cystic fibrosis." *Journal of Pediatrics*, 122: 810–812, 1993.

National Research Council. *Diet and Health: Implications For Reducing Chronic Disease Risk*. Washington, DC: National Academy Press, 1989.

Nordstrom, J. "Trace mineral nutrition in the elderly." *American Journal of Clinical Nutrition*, 36: 788–795, 1982.

Ornish, D. "Can lifestyle changes reverse coronary heart disease?" *Lancet*, 336: 129–133, 1990.

Oyama, Y. "Myricetin and quercetin, the flavonoid constituents of Ginkgo biloba extract, greatly reduce oxidative metabolism in both resting and Ca(2+)-loaded brain neurons." *Brain Research*, 635(1–2): 125–129, 1994.

Paolisso, G. "Chronic intake of pharmacological doses of vitamin E might be useful in the therapy of elderly patients with coronary heart disease." *American Journal of Clinical Nutrition*, 61: 848–852, 1995.

Parker, L. "Alpha Lipoic Acid as a biological antioxidant." *Free Radical Medicine*, 19(2): 227–250, 1995.

Parkinson Study Group. "DATATOP: A multicenter controlled clinical trial in early Parkinson's disease." *Archives in Neurology*, 46: 1052–1060, 1989.

Pascale, A. "Protein kinase C activation and anti-amnesic effect of acetylcarnitine in *in vitro* and *in vivo* studies." *European Journal of Pharmacology*, 256(1–2): 1–7, 1994.

Pettigrew, J. "Clinical and neurochemical effects of acetyl-l-carnitine in Alzheimer's disease." *Neurobiology of Aging*, 16: 1–4, 1995.

Rai, A. "A double-blind, placebo-controlled study of Ginkgo biloba extract ('Tanakan') in elderly outpatients with mild to moderate memory impairment." *Current Medical Research Opinion*, 12: 350–355, 1991.

Ramassamy, C. "Prevention by a Ginkgo biloba extract (GBE 761) of the dopaminergic neurotoxicity of MPTP." *Journal of Pharmacy and Pharmacology*, 42(11): 785–789, 1990.

Rosadini, G. "Phosphatidylserine: Quantitative EEG Effects in Healthy Volunteers." *Neuropsychobiology*, 24: 42–48, 1990–1991.

Salvioli, G. "L-acetylcarnitine treatment of mental decline in the elderly." *Drugs Under Experimental and Clinical Research*, 20(4): 169–176, 1994.

Schmidt, E. "Omega-3 fatty acids. Current status in cardiovascular medicine." *Drugs*, 47: 405–424, 1994.

Scott, B. "Lipoic and dihydrolipoic acids as antioxidants: A critical evaluation." *Free Radical Research*, 20: 119–133, 1994.

Seidelin, K. "N-3 fatty acids in adipose tissue and coronary artery disease are inversely correlated." *American Journal of Clinical Nutrition*, 55: 1117–1119, 1992.

Spagnoli, A. "Long-term acetyl-L-carnitine treatment in Alzheimer's disease." *Neurology*, 41: 1726–1732, 1991.

Stewart, J. "Low B_6 levels in depressed outpatients." *Biological Psychiatry*, 19(4): 613–616, 1984.

Suzuki, Y. "Alpha-lipoic acid is a potent inhibitor of NF-kB activation in human T cells." *Biochemical Biophysical Research Communication,* 189: 1709–1715, 1992.

Takagi, Y. "Calcium treatment of essential hypertension in elderly patients evaluated by 24 H monitoring." *American Journal of Hypertension,* 4: 836–839, 1991.

Tam, S. "Mesoprefrontal dopaminergic neurons: Can tyrosine availability influence their functions?" *Biochemical Pharmacology,* 53(4): 441–453, 1997.

Turlapaty, P. "Magnesium deficiency produces spasms of coronary arteries: Relationship to etiology of sudden death ischemic heart disease." *Science,* 208: 199–200, 1980.

Valenzuela, A. "Silymarin protection against hepatic lipid peroxidation induced by acute ethanol intoxication in the rat." *Biological Pharmacology,* 34(12): 2209–2212, 1985.

Young, S. "Folic acid and psychopathology." *Progress in Neuropsychopharmacology and Biological Psychiatry,* 13: 841–863, 1989.

Young, S. "Some effects of dietary components (amino acids, carbohydrate, folic acid) on brain serotonin synthesis, mood, and behavior." *Canadian Journal of Physiology and Pharmacology,* 69: 893–903, 1989.

Chapter 7 "Smart" Drugs

Aguglia, E. "Comparison of teniloxazine and piracetam in Alzheimer-type or vascular dementia." *Current Therapeutic Research,* 56(3): 250–257, 1995.

Birge, S. "Is there a role for estrogen replacement therapy in the prevention and treatment of dementia?" *American Geriatrics Society,* 44(7): 865–870, 1996.

Branconnier, R. "The efficacy of the cerebral metabolic enhancers in the treatment of senile dementia." *Psychopharmacology Bulletin,* 19(2): 212–220, 1983.

Cumin, R. "Effects of the novel compound aniracetam (RO13-5057) upon impaired learning and memory in rodents." *Psychopharmacology,* 78: 104–111, 1982.

Dean, W. *Smart Drugs II: The Next Generation.* Petaluma, CA: Smart Publications, p. 287, 1993.

Deberdt, W. "Interaction between psychological and pharmacological treatment in cognitive impairment." *Life Sciences,* 55(25–26): 2057–2066, 1994.

"Effect of deprenyl on the progression of disability in early Parkinson's disease." *New England Journal of Medicine,* 321: 1364–1371, 1989.

Ferrero, E. "Controlled clinical trial of oxiracetam in the treatment of chronic cerebrovascular insufficiency in the elderly." *Current Therapeutic Research,* 36(2): 298–308, 1984.

Finkel, M. "Phenytoin revisited." *Journal of Clinical Therapeutics,* 6(5): 577–591, 1984.

Gibbs, M. "Diphenylhydantoin extension of short-term and intermediate stages of memory." *Behavior and Brain Research,* 11(2): 203–208, 1984.

Groo, D. "Comparison of the effects of vinpocetine, vincamine, and nicergoline on the normal and hypoxia damaged learning process in spontaneously hypertensive rats." *Drug Development Research,* 15: 75–85, 1988.

Loriaux, S. "The effects of nicotinic acid (niacin) and xanthinol nicotinate on human memory in different categories of age, a double blind study." *Psychopharmacology,* 87: 390–395, 1985.

Nagy, I. "Electron spin resonance spectroscopic demonstration of the hydroxyl free radical scavenger properties of dimethylaminoethanol in spin trapping experiments confirming the molecular basis for the biological effects of centrophenoxine." *Archives of Gerontology and Geriatrics,* 3(4): 297–310, 1984.

Pilch, H. "Piracetam elevates muscarinic cholinergic receptor density in the frontal cortex of aged but not of young mice." *Psychopharmacology,* 94: 74–78, 1988.

Poschel, B. "Pharmacology underlying the cognition-activating properties of pramiracetam (CI-879)." *Psychopharmacology Bulletin,* 19(4): 720–721, 1983.

Thienhaus, O. "A controlled double-blind study of high-dose dihy-droergotoxine mesylate (Hydergine) in mild dementia." *Journal of American Geriatric Society,* 35(3): 219–223, March 1987.

Tollefson, G. "Short-term effects of the calcium channel blocker nimodipine (Bay-e-9736) in the management of primary degenerative dementia." *Biological Psychiatry,* 27(10): 1133–1142, 1990.

Stroescu, V. "The Experimental and Clinical Pharmacology of Procaine, Gerovital H3 and Aslavital." *Romanian Journal of Gerontology and Geriatrics,* 9(4): 427–437, 1988.

Yamazaki, N. "Idebenone improves learning and memory impairment induced by cholinergic or serotonergic dysfunction in rats." *Archives of Gerontology and Geriatrics,* 8(3): 225–239, 1989.

Chapter 8 Chelation and Oxygen Therapies

Altman, N. *Oxygen Healing Therapies.* Rochester, Vermont: Healing Arts Press, 1995.

Blummer, W. "Ninety percent reduction in cancer mortality after chelation therapy with EDTA." *Journal of Advancement in Medicine,* 2(1, 2): 183–188, 1989.

Casdorph, H., and M. Walker. *Toxic Metal Syndrome.* Garden City Park, NY: Avery Publishing Group, 1995.

Cranton, E. *Bypassing Bypass.* Troutdale, VA: Hampton Roads Publishers, 1990.

Devesa, E. "Ozone therapy in ischemic cerebrovascular disease." *Ozone in Medicine: Proceedings of the Eleventh Ozone World Congress,* Stamford, CT, International Ozone Association, Pan American Committee, M–4–10–18, 1993.

Farr, C. *Protocol for the Intravenous Administration of Hydrogen Peroxide.* Oklahoma City: International Bio-Oxidative Medicine Foundation, 29–31, 1993.

Halstead, B. *The Scientific Basis of EDTA Chelation.* Colton, CA: Golden Quill Publishers, Inc., 1979.

Kramer, F. "Ozone in the dental practice." In *Medical Applications of Ozone,* Julius LaRaus, editor, Norwalk, CT: International Ozone Association, Pan American Committee, 258–265, 1983.

Lin, D. *Free Radicals and Disease Prevention.* New Canaan, CT: Keats Publishing, p. 79, 1993.

McCabe, E. *Oxygen Therapies.* Morrisville, NY: Energy Publications, 1988.

Rodriquez, M. "Ozone therapy for senile dementia." *Ozone in Medicine: Proceedings of the Eleventh Ozone World Congress,* Stamford, CT: International Ozone Association, Pan American Committee, M–4–9–25, 1993.

Rudolph, C. "A nonsurgical approach to obstructive carotid stenosis using EDTA chelation." *Journal of Advancement in Medicine,* 4(3): 157–168, 1991.

Setty, B. "Effects of hydrogen peroxide on vascular arachidonic acid metabolism." *Prostaglandins, Leukotrienes and Medicine,* 14: 205–213, 1984.

Shilling. C. *Underwater Medicine and Related Sciences: A Guide to the Literature.* New York: Plenum Publications, Volume 2, 1975.

Sunnen, G. "Ozone in medicine: overview and future direction." *Journal of Advancement in Medicine,* 1(3), 1988.

Trowbridge, J. *The Healing Powers of Chelation Therapy.* Stamford, CT: New Way of Life, Inc., 1992.

Chapter 9 NAET, Niacin Detox Saunas, and Fasting

Cutler, E. *Winning the War Against Asthma & Allergies.* Albany, NY: Delmar Publishers, 1997.

Nambudripad, D. *Say Goodbye to Illness.* Buena Park, CA: Delta Publishing, 1993.

Randolph, T. *An Alternate Approach to Environmental Illness.* New York: Harper & Row, 1989.

Roehm, D. "Effects of a program of sauna baths and megavitamins on adipose DDE and PCBs and on clearing of symptoms of agent orange (Dioxin) toxicity." *Clinical Research,* 31: 243, 1983.

Root, D. "Diagnosis and treatment of patients presenting subclinical signs and symptoms of exposure to chemicals which bioaccumulate in human tissue." Proceedings of the National Conference on Hazardous Wastes and Environmental Emergencies, Hazardous Materials Control Research Institute, 1985.

Root, D. "The biotoxic reduction program: eliminating body pollution." *The Townsend Letter for Doctors,* (46), February 1987.

Schnare, D. "Reductions of hexachlorobenzene and polychlorinated biphenyl human body burdens." International Agency for Research on Cancer, World Health Organization, Publication Series, Volume 77, Oxford University Press, 1985.

Bibliography

Abalan, F. "B-12 deficiency in presenile dementia." *Biological Psychiatry*, 20: 1247–1251, 1985.

Abu-Shakra, M. "Parasitic infectional autoimmunity." *Autoimmunity*, 9(4): 337–344, 1991.

Ackerman, S. *Discovering the Brain.* Washington, DC: The National Academy Press, 1992.

Aggleton, J., editor. *The Amygdala.* New York: Wiley-Liss, 1992.

Aguglia, E. "Comparison of teniloxazine and piracetam in Alzheimer-type or vascular dementia." *Current Therapeutic Research*, 56(3): 250–257, 1995.

Albertson, T. "The effect of lindane and long-term potentiation (LTP) on pyramidal cell excitability in the rat hippocampal slice." *Neuro Toxicology*, 18(2): 469–478, 1997.

Altman, N. *Oxygen Healing Therapies.* Rochester, Vermont: Healing Arts Press, 1995.

"Alzheimer's alchemy." *Science News*, 141: 152–153, March 7, 1992.

Anderson, A. "Neurotoxic follies." *Psychology Today*, 30–42, July 1982.

Arendt, T. "Impairment in memory function and neurodegenerative changes in the cholinergic basal forebrain system induced by chronic intake of ethanol." *Journal of Neural Transmission*, Supplementum 44: 173–187, 1994.

Ashford, N. *Chemical Exposures.* New York: Van Nostrand Reinhold, 1991.

Avdulov, N. "Amyloid beta-peptides increase annular and bulk fluidity and induce lipid peroxidation in brain synaptic plasma membranes." *Journal of Neurochemistry,* 68(5): 2086–2091, 1991.

Balch, James F., and Phyllis A. Balch. *Prescription for Nutritional Healing,* 2nd edition. Garden City Park, NY: Avery Publishing Group, 1997.

Ballinger, S. "Mitochondrial DNA may hold a key to human degenerative diseases." *Journal of the National Institutes of Health Research,* 4: 62–66, 1992.

Barbiroli, B. "Lipoic (thiotic) acid increases brain energy availability and skeletal muscle performance as shown by in vivo 31P-MRS in a patient with mitochondria cytopathy." *Journal of Neurology,* 242 (7): 472–477, 1995.

Baxter, M. "Intact spatial learning following lesions of basal forebrain cholinergic neurons." *Neuroreport,* 7(8): 1417–20, 1996.

Bechara, A. "Failure to respond autonomically to anticipated future outcomes following damage to prefrontal cortex." *Cerebral Cortex,* 6(2): 215–225, 1996.

Becker, R. *Cross Currents: The Perils of Electropollution, The Promise of Electromedicine.* New York: Jeremy P. Tarcher, 1990.

Bellinger, D. "Longitudinal analyses of prenatal and postnatal lead exposure and early cognitive development." *New England Journal of Medicine,* 316: 1037–1043, 1987.

Benjamin, J. "Inositol treatment in psychiatry." *Psychopharmacology Bulletin,* 31: 167–175, 1995.

Benton, D. "The impact of selenium supplementation on mood." *Biological Psychiatry,* 29: 1092–1098, 1991.

Birge, S. "Is there a role for estrogen replacement therapy in the prevention and treatment of dementia?" *American Geriatrics Society,* 44(7): 865–870, 1996.

Blaylock, R. *Excitotoxins: The Taste That Kills.* Santa Fe, NM: Health Press, 1997.

Blummer, W. "Ninety percent reduction in cancer mortality after chelation therapy with EDTA." *Journal of Advancement in Medicine,* 2(1, 2): 183–188, 1989.

Bonavita, E. "Study of the efficacy and tolerability of L-acetylcarnitine therapy in the senile brain." *International Journal of Clinical Pharmacology Therapy and Toxicology,* 24: 511–516, 1986.

Borgstrom, L. "Pharmacokinetics of N-acetylcysteine in man." *European Journal of Clinical Pharmacology,* 31: 271–272, 1986.

Branconnier, R. "The efficacy of the cerebral metabolic enhancers in the treatment of senile dementia." *Psychopharmacology Bulletin,* 19(2): 212–220, 1983.

Bull, I. "Vitamin B-12 and folate status in acute geropsychiatric inpatients." *Nutrition Report,* 9(1): 1, 1991.

Burnet, F. "A possible role of zinc in the pathology of dementia." *Lancet,* I: 186–188, 1981.

Butterworth, R. "Effects of thiamine deficiency on brain metabolism: Implications for the pathogenesis of Wernicke-Korsakoff syndrome." *Alcohol Alcoholism,* 24: 271–279, 1989.

Calkin, R. *Perfumery.* New York: John Wiley and Sons, Inc., 1994.

Calvani, M. "Action of acetyl-l-carnitine in neurodegeneration and Alzheimer's disease." *Annals of the New York Academy of Science,* 663: 483–486, 1992.

Cantz, D. "Lecithin and choline in human health and disease." *Nutrition Reviews,* 52(10): 327–339, 1994.

Carney, M. "Thiamin, riboflavin and pyridoxine deficiency in psychiatric in-patients." *British Journal of Psychiatry,* 141: 271–272, 1982.

_____. "Vitamin deficiency and mental symptoms." *British Journal of Psychiatry,* 156: 878–882, 1990.

Casdorph, H., and M. Walker. *Toxic Metal Syndrome.* Garden City Park, NY: Avery Publishing Group, 1995.

Chernoff, R. "Nutrition and aging," in Shils, M. *Modern Nutrition in Health and Disease.* Philadelphia: Lea & Febinger, 1988.

Christensen, L. "The role of caffeine and sugar in depression." *Nutrition Report,* 9(3): 17–24, 1991.

Chui, H. "Extrapyramidal signs and psychiatric symptoms predict faster cognitive decline in Alzheimer's disease." *Archives of Neurology,* 51(7): 676–681, 1994.

Cichoke, Anthony J. *The Complete Book of Enzyme Therapy.* Garden City Park, NY: Avery Publishing Group, 1999.

Conn, M., editor. *Neuroscience in Medicine.* Philadelphia: J. B. Lippincott Company, 1995.

Consumer Product Safety Commission. "1990 Product Summary Report: National Electronic Injury Surveillance System." Washington, DC: National Injury Information Clearinghouse, 1990.

Cranton, E. *Bypassing Bypass.* Troutdale, VA: Hampton Roads Publishers, 1990.

Crawley, J. "Biological actions of cholecystokinin." *Peptides,* 15(4): 731–55, 1994.

Crissinger, K. "Pathophysiology of gastrointestinal mucosal permeability." *Journal of Internal Medicine,* 228(1): 145–154, 1990.

Crook, Thomas. Interview, March 15, 1998.

Cumin, R. "Effects of the novel compound aniracetam (RO13-5057) upon impaired learning and memory in rodents." *Psychopharmacology,* 78: 104–111, 1982.

Cutler, E. *Winning the War Against Asthma & Allergies,* Albany, NY: Delmar Publishers, 1997.

Dadd, D. *Nontoxic, Natural, and Earthwise,* New York: St. Martin's Press, 1990.

Davis, S. "Acetyl-L-carnitine: behavioral, electrophysiological, and neurochemical effects." *Neurobiology of Aging,* 14(1): 107–115, 1993.

Dean, W. *Smart Drugs II: The Next Generation.* Petaluma, CA: Smart Publications, 1993.

Deberdt, W. "Interaction between psychological and pharmacological treatment in cognitive impairment." *Life Sciences,* 55(25–26): 2057–2066, 1994.

Demitrack, M. "Relation of dissociative phenomena to levels of cerebrospinal fluid monoamine metabolites and beta-endorphin in patients with eating disorders: A pilot study." *Psychiatry Research,* 49(1): 1–10, 1993.

Devesa, E. "Ozone therapy in ischemic cerebrovascular disease." *Ozone in Medicine: Proceedings of the Eleventh Ozone World Congress,* Stamford, CT, International Ozone Association, Pan American Committee, M–4–10–18, 1993.

Dexter, D. "Basal lipid-peroxidation in substantia nigra is increased in Parkinson's disease." 52: 381–389, 1989.

Didier, M. "Chronic glutamate toxicity causes DNA damage." *Neurology,* 44: A236, 1994.

"Effect of deprenyl on the progression of disability in early Parkinson's disease." *New England Journal of Medicine,* 321: 1364–1371, 1989.

Elman, J. "Learning and development in neural networks: the importance of starting small." *Cognition,* 48(1): 71–99, 1993.

Environmental Protection Agency. "Suspended, canceled, and restricted pesticides." Washington, DC: Government Printing Office, February 1990.

"Export of pesticides is not adequately monitored by EPA." General Accounting Office, Washington, DC: GAO/RCED 89–126, 1989.

Farr, C. *Protocol for the Intravenous Administration of Hydrogen Peroxide.* Oklahoma City: International Bio-Oxidative Medicine Foundation, 1993.

Ferrero, E. "Controlled clinical trial of oxiracetam in the treatment of chronic cerebrovascular insufficiency in the elderly." *Current Therapeutic Research,* 36(2): 298–308, 1984.

Feychting, M. "Dementia and occupational exposure to magnetic fields." *Scandinavian Journal of Work, Environment and Health,* 1998.

Fincher, C. *Healthy Living in a Toxic World.* Colorado Springs, CO: Pinon Press, 1996.

Finkel, M. "Phenytoin revisited." *Journal of Clinical Therapeutics,* 6(5): 577–591, 1984.

Fisher, A. "Adverse nail reactions and paresthesia from 'photo-bonded acrylate sculptured nails.'" *Cutis,* 45: 293–94, 1990.

Frizel, D. "Plasma calcium and magnesium in depression." *British Journal of Psychiatry,* 115: 1375–1377, 1969.

Fulder, Stephen. *The Ginseng Book.* Garden City Park, NY: Avery Publishing Group, 1996.

Galland, L. "Intestinal protozoan infection is a common unsuspected cause of chronic illness." *Journal of Advanced Medicine,* 2: 539–552, 1989.

Ghadirian, A. "Folic acid deficiency and depression." *Psychosomatics,* 21(11): 926–929, 1980.

Gibbs, M. "Diphenylhydantoin extension of short-term and intermediate stages of memory." *Behavior and Brain Research,* 11(2): 203–208, 1984.

Glick, J. "Dementia: the role of magnesium deficiency and an hypothesis concerning the pathogenesis of Alzheimer's disease." *Medical Hypothesis,* 31: 211–225, 1991.

Golan, R. *Optimal Wellness.* New York: Ballantine Books, 1995.

Grady, C. "Age-related reductions in human recognition memory due to impaired encoding." *Science,* 269 (5221): 218–221, 1995.

Grobbee, D. "Coffee, caffeine, and cardiovascular disease in men." *New England Journal of Medicine,* 323(15): 1026–1032, 1990.

Groo, D. "Comparison of the effects of vinpocetine, vincamine, and nicergoline on the normal and hypoxia damaged learning process in spontaneously hypertensive rats." *Drug Development Research,* 15: 75–85, 1988.

Hallenbeck, W. *Pesticides and Human Health.* New York: Springer-Verlag, 1985.

Halliwell, B. "Antioxidants in human health and disease." *Annual Review of Nutrition,* 16: 33–50, 1996.

Halstead, B. *The Scientific Basis of EDTA Chelation.* Colton, CA: Golden Quill Publishers, Inc., 1979.

Harbige, L. "Nutrition and immunity with emphasis on infection and autoimmune disease." *Nutrition and Health,* 10(4): 285–312, 1996.

Harik, S. "Altered glucose metabolism in microvessels from patients with Alzheimer's disease." *Annals of Neurobiology*, 26: 91–94, 1991.

Hayes, W. *Pesticides Studied In Man*. Baltimore, MD: Williams and Wilkins, 1982.

Hershey, L. "Dementia associated with stroke." *Stroke*, 21: 9–11, 1990.

Huxtable, R. "The pharmacology of extinction." *Journal of Ethnopharmacology*, 37(1): 1–11, 1992.

Jacobson, J. "Evidence for PCBs as neurodevelopmental toxicants in humans." *Neurotoxicology*, 18(2): 415–425, 1997.

Jahnke, A. "Into the mouths of babes." *Psychology Today*, 26: 8, 1993.

Jenkins, A. "Do non-steroidal anti-inflammatory drugs increase colonic permeability?" *Gut*, 32: 66–69, 1991.

Jeyaratnam, J. "Acute pesticide poisoning: a major global health problem." *World Health Statistics Quarterly*, 43(3): 139–144, 1990.

Kalaria, R. "Serum amyloid P in Alzheimer's disease: Implications for dysfunction of the blood brain barrier." *Annals New York Academy of Science*, 640: 145–148, 1991.

Kandel, E. *Essentials of Neural Science and Behavior*. Stamford, CT: Appellation & Lane, 1995.

Kleijnen, J. "Ginkgo biloba for cerebral insufficiency." *British Journal of Clinical Pharmacology*, 34: 352–358, 1992.

Klein-Schwartz, W. "Agricultural and horticultural chemical poisoning: mortality and morbidity in the United States." *Annals of Emergency Medicine*, 29(2): 232–8, 1997.

Kolata, G. "Studies find brain grows new cells." *The New York Times*, B9, B12, March 17, 1998.

Kramer, F. "Ozone in the dental practice." In *Medical Applications of Ozone*, Julius LaRaus, editor, Norwalk, CT: International Ozone Association, Pan American Committee, 258–265, 1983.

Laakso, M. "MRI of amygdala fails to diagnose early Alzheimer's disease." *Neuroreport*, 6(17): 2414–2418, 1995.

Lai, H. "Acute exposure to a 60-Hz magnetic field affects rats' performance in the water maze performance." *Bioelectromagnetics,* 19: 117–122, 1998.

_____. "Acute exposure to a 60-Hz magnetic field increases DNA single-strand breaks in rat brain cells." *Bioelectromagnetics,* 18: 156–165, 1997.

_____. "Effects of a 60-Hz magnetic field on central cholinergic systems of the rat." *Bioelectromagnetics,* 14: 5–15, 1993.

_____. "Melatonin and a spin-trap compound blocked radio frequency radiation-induced DNA single and double strand breaks in rat brain cells." *Journal of Pineal Research,* 22: 151–162, 1997.

Langley, W. "Central nervous system magnesium deficiency." *Archives of International Medicine,* 151: 593–596, 1991.

Leaf, A. "Cardiovascular effects of omega-3 fatty acids." *New England Journal of Medicine,* 318: 549–557.

Levenstein, M.K. *Everyday Cancer Risks and How to Avoid Them.* Garden City Park, NY: Avery Publishing Group, 1992.

Levi, S. "Increased energy expenditure in Parkinson's disease." *British Medical Journal,* 301: 1256–1257, 1990.

Levitt, B. *Electromagnetic Fields: A Consumer's Guide to the Issues and How to Protect Ourselves.* New York: Harcourt Brace & Company, 1995.

Lewis, D. "Intracellular regulation of ion channels in cell membranes." *Mayo Clinic Proceedings,* 65: 1127–1143, 1990.

Lifton, B. *Bug Busters.* Garden City Park, NY: Avery Publishing Group, 1991.

Lin, D. *Free Radicals and Disease Prevention.* New Canaan, CT: Keats Publishing, 1993.

Loriaux, S. "The effects of nicotinic acid (niacin) and xanthinol nicotinate on human memory in different categories of age, a double blind study." *Psychopharmacology,* 87: 390–395, 1985.

Lussi, A. "The amalgam problems: Recommendations on patient assessment and counseling." *Schwizerische Medizinische Wochenschrift,* 127(10): 398–405, 1997.

Lyras, L. "An assessment of oxidative damage to proteins, lipids, and DNA in brain from patients with Alzheimer's disease." *Journal of Neurochemistry*, 68(5): 2061–2169, 1997.

Mackay, S. "Regional gray and white matter metabolite differences in subjects with AD, with subcortical ischemic vascular dementia, and elderly controls with 1H magnetic resonance spectroscopic imaging." *Archives of Neurology*, 53(2): 167–174, 1996.

Malt, U. "Physical and mental problems attributed to dental amalgam fillings: A descriptive study of 99 self-referred patients compared to 272 controls." *Psychosomatic Medicine*, 59(1): 32–41, 1997.

Marks, J. *Contact and Occupational Dermatology*. St. Louis, MO: Mosby Year Book, 1992.

McCabe, E. *Oxygen Therapies*. Morrisville, NY: Energy Publications, 1988.

McConnachie, P. "Immune alterations in humans exposed to the termiticide technical chlordane." *Archives of Environmental Health*, 27: 296–297, 1992.

McEntee, W. "Glutamate: Its role in learning, memory, and the aging brain." *Psychopharmacology*, 111(4): 391–401, 1993.

McGeer, P. "The inflammatory response system of the brain: Implications for therapy of Alzheimer and other neurodegenerative diseases." *Brain Research Reviews*, 21: 195–218, 1995.

McMahan, S. "Depressive symptomatology in women and residential proximity to high-voltage transmission lines." *American Journal of Epidemiology*, 139: 58–63, 1994.

Meister, T., editor. *Farm Chemicals Handbook*. Willoughby, Ohio: Meister Publishing Company, 1990.

Merck Manual of Medical Information, The. Whitehouse Station, NJ: Merck Research Laboratories, 1997.

Mindell, E. *Vitamin Bible*. New York: Warner Books, 1991.

Misra, U. "A study of cognitive functions in methyl-iso-cyanate victims one year after Bhopal accident." *Neuro Toxicology*, 18(2): 381–386, 1997.

Moon, C. "Main and interaction effects of metallic pollutants on cognitive functioning." *Journal of Learning Disabilities*, 18(4): 217–221, 1985.

Mooradian, A. "The effect of aging on the blood-brain barrier. A review." *Neurobiological Aging*, 9: 31–39, 1988.

Murray, J. "Aluminum neurotoxicity: a re-evaluation." *Clinical Neuropharmacology*, 14: 179–185, 1991.

Murray, M. *Encyclopedia of Nutritional Supplements*. Rocklin, CA: Prima Publishing, 1996.

Nagamatsu, M. "Lipoic acid improves nerve blood flow, reduces oxidative stress, and improves distal nerve conduction in experimental diabetic neuropathy." *Diabetes Care*, 18: 1160–1167, 1995.

Nagy, I. "Electron spin resonance spectroscopic demonstration of the hydroxyl free radical scavenger properties of dimethylaminoethanol in spin trapping experiments confirming the molecular basis for the biological effects of centrophenoxine." *Archives of Gerontology and Geriatrics*, 3(4): 297–310, 1984.

Nambudripad, D. *Say Goodbye to Illness*. Buena Park, CA: Delta Publishing, 1993.

Nasr, S. "Correction of vitamin E deficiency with fat-soluble versus water-miscible preparations of vitamin E in patients with cystic fibrosis." *Journal of Pediatrics*, 122: 810–812, 1993.

National Research Council. *Diet and Health: Implications For Reducing Chronic Disease Risk*. Washington, DC: National Academy Press, 1989.

National Research Council. *Toxicity Testing, Strategies to Determine Needs and Priorities*. Washington, DC: National Academy Press, 1984.

New Chemicals Program. United States Environmental Protection Agency, Office of Pollution Prevention and Toxics, EPA–734–F–95–001, May 13, 1995.

Nordstrom, J. "Trace mineral nutrition in the elderly." *American Journal of Clinical Nutrition*, 36: 788–795, 1982.

Novelli, J. "Glutamate becomes neurotoxic via the N-methyl-D-aspartate receptor when intracellular energy levels are reduced." *Brain Research*, 451: 205–212, 1988.

Ornish, D. "Can lifestyle changes reverse coronary heart disease?" *Lancet*, 336: 129–133, 1990.

Oscar-Berman, M. "Association learning and recognition memory in alcoholic Korsakoff patients." *Neuropsychology*, 2: 282–289, 1997.

Oskarsson, A. "Total and inorganic mercury in breast milk and blood in relation to fish consumption and amalgam fillings in lactating women." *Archives of Environmental Health*, 51(3): 234–241, 1996.

Otamiri, T. "Ginkgo biloba extract prevents mucosal damage associated with small-intestinal ischaemia." *Scandinavian Journal of Gastroenterology*, 24: 666–670, 1989.

Oyama, Y. "Myricetin and quercetin, the flavonoid constituents of Ginkgo biloba extract, greatly reduce oxidative metabolism in both resting and Ca(2+)-loaded brain neurons." *Brain Research*, 635(1–2): 125–129, 1994.

Paolisso, G. "Chronic intake of pharmacological doses of vitamin E might be useful in the therapy of elderly patients with coronary heart disease." *American Journal of Clinical Nutrition*, 61: 848–852, 1995.

Parent, A. *Carpenter's Human Neuroanatomy*, 9th edition. Baltimore: Williams & Wilkins, 1996.

Parker, L. "Alpha Lipoic Acid as a biological antioxidant." *Free Radical Medicine*, 19(2): 227–250, 1995.

Parkinson Study Group. "DATATOP: A multicenter controlled clinical trial in early Parkinson's disease." *Archives in Neurology*, 46: 1052–1060, 1989.

Pascale, A. "Protein kinase C activation and anti-amnesic effect of acetylcarnitine in *in vitro* and *in vivo* studies." *European Journal of Pharmacology*, 256(1–2): 1–7, 1994.

Pettigrew, J. "Clinical and neurochemical effects of acetyl-l-carnitine in Alzheimer's disease." *Neurobiology of Aging*, 16: 1–4, 1995.

Pilch, H. "Piracetam elevates muscarinic cholinergic receptor density in the frontal cortex of aged but not of young mice." *Psychopharmacology*, 94: 74–78, 1988.

Poole, C. "Depressive symptoms and headaches in relation to proximity to an alternating-current transmission line right-of-way." *American Journal of Epidemiology*, 137: 318–330, 1993.

Poschel, B. "Pharmacology underlying the cognition-activating properties of pramiracetam (CI-879)." *Psychopharmacology Bulletin*, 19(4): 720–721, 1983.

Rai, A. "A double-blind, placebo-controlled study of Ginkgo biloba extract ('Tanakan') in elderly outpatients with mild to moderate memory impairment." *Current Medical Research Opinion*, 12: 350–355, 1991.

Ramassamy, C. "Prevention by a Ginkgo biloba extract (GBE 761) of the dopaminergic neurotoxicity of MPTP." *Journal of Pharmacy and Pharmacology*, 42(11): 785–789, 1990.

Randolph, T. *An Alternate Approach to Environmental Illness*. New York: Harper & Row, 1989.

_____. *An Alternative Approach to Allergies*. New York: Harper & Row, 1989.

Rapp. P. "Preserved neuron number in the hippocampus of aged rats with spatial learning deficits." *Proceedings of the National Academy of Sciences of the United States of America*, 93(18): 9926–9930, 1996.

Ratcliffe, H. "Human exposure to mercury: A critical assessment of the evidence of adverse health effects. *Journal of Toxicology and Environmental Health*, 49(3): 221–270, 1996.

Reisberg, B. *Alzheimer's Disease: The Standard Reference*. New York: Free Press, 1983.

_____. "Dementia staging in chronic care populations." *Alzheimer's Disease and Associated Disorders*, vol 8(1): S188–205, 1994.

Reiter, R. "Alterations of the circadian melatonin rhythm by the electromagnetic spectrum: a study in environmental toxicology." *Regulatory Toxicology and Pharmacology*, 15: 226–244, 1992.

Robinson, T. "Effects of cortical serotonin depletion induced by 3, 4-methylenedioxymethamphetamine (MDMA) on behavior, before and after additional cholinergic blockade." *Neuropsychopharmacology*, 8(1): 77–85, 1993.

Rodriquez, M. "Ozone therapy for senile dementia." *Ozone in Medicine: Proceedings of the Eleventh Ozone World Congress,* Stamford, CT: International Ozone Association, Pan American Committee, M–4–9–25, 1993.

Roehm, D. "Effects of a program of sauna baths and megavitamins on adipose DDE and PCBs and on clearing of symptoms of agent orange (Dioxin) toxicity." *Clinical Research,* 31: 243, 1983.

Root, D. "The biotoxic reduction program: eliminating body pollution." *The Townsend Letter for Doctors,* (46), February 1987.

_____. "Diagnosis and treatment of patients presenting subclinical signs and symptoms of exposure to chemicals which bioaccumulate in human tissue." Proceedings of the National Conference on Hazardous Wastes and Environmental Emergencies, Hazardous Materials Control Research Institute, 1985.

Rosadini, G. "Phosphatidylserine: Quantitative EEG Effects in Healthy Volunteers." *Neuropsychobiology,* 24: 42–48, 1990–1991.

Rowland, A. "The effect of occupational exposure to mercury vapor on the fertility of female dental assistants." *Occupational and Environmental Medicine,* 51(1): 28–34, 1994.

Rudolph, C. "A nonsurgical approach to obstructive carotid stenosis using EDTA chelation." *Journal of Advancement in Medicine,* 4(3): 157–168, 1991.

Rugg, M. "Differential activation of the prefrontal cortex in successful and unsuccessful memory retrieval." *Brain,* 119(6): 2073–2083, 1996.

Salvioli, G. "L-acetylcarnitine treatment of mental decline in the elderly." *Drugs Under Experimental and Clinical Research,* 20(4): 169–176, 1994.

Sayre, L. "4-Hydroxynonenal-derived advanced lipid peroxidation end products are increased in Alzheimer's disease." *Journal of Neurochemistry,* 6(5): 2092–2097, 1997.

Schapira, A. "Mitochondrial complex I deficiency in Parkinson's disease." *Journal of Neurochemistry,* 54: 823–827, 1990.

Scheibel, A. "Alzheimer's disease as a capillary dementia." *Annals of Medicine,* 21: 103–107, 1989.

Schmidt, E. "Omega-3 fatty acids. Current status in cardiovascular medicine." *Drugs*, 47: 405–424, 1994.

Schnare, D. "Reductions of hexachlorobenzene and polychlorinated biphenyl human body burdens." International Agency for Research on Cancer, World Health Organization, Publication Series, Volume 77, Oxford University Press, 1985.

Schwartz, G. *In Bad Taste: The MSG Syndrome.* Sante Fe, NM: Health Press, 1988.

Scott, B. "Lipoic and dihydrolipoic acids as antioxidants: A critical evaluation." *Free Radical Research,* 20: 119–133, 1994.

Sehnert, K. "Is mercury toxicity an autoimmune disorder?" *Townsend Letter for Doctors & Patients,* 134–137, October, 1995.

Seidelin, K. "N-3 fatty acids in adipose tissue and coronary artery disease are inversely correlated." *American Journal of Clinical Nutrition,* 55: 1117–1119, 1992.

Setty, B. "Effects of hydrogen peroxide on vascular arachidonic acid metabolism." *Prostaglandins, Leukotrienes and Medicine,* 14: 205–213, 1984.

Shilling. C. *Underwater Medicine and Related Sciences: A Guide to the Literature.* New York: Plenum Publications, Volume 2, 1975.

Siegal, G., editor. *Basic Neurochemistry.* New York: Raven Press, 1989.

Siesjo, B. "Calcium, excitotoxins, and neuronal death in the brain." *Annals of the New York Academy of Sciences,* 568: 234–251, 1989.

Singer, R. *Neurotoxicity Guidebook.* New York: Van Nostrand Reinhold, 1990.

Small, G. "Age-associated memory loss: initial neuropsychological and cerebral metabolic findings of a longitudinal study." *International Psychogeriatrics,* 6(1): 23–44, 1994.

_____. "Predictors of cognitive change in middle-aged and older adults with memory loss." *American Journal of Psychiatry,* 152(12): 1757–1764, 1995.

Sobel, E. "Electromagnetic field exposure may cause increased production of amyloid beta and eventually lead to Alzheimer's disease." *Neurology,* 47: 1594–1600, 1996.

Spagnoli, A. "Long-term acetyl-L-carnitine treatment in Alzheimer's disease." *Neurology*, 41: 1726–1732, 1991.

Steinman, D. *Living Healthy in a Toxic World.* New York: The Berkley Publishing Group, 1996.

_____. *The Safe Shopper's Bible.* New York: MacMillan Publishing, 1995.

Stewart, J. "Low B-6 levels in depressed outpatients." *Biological Psychiatry*, 19(4): 613–616, 1984.

_____. "Patch testing to cosmetics and topical drugs." *American Journal of Contact Dermatitis*, 7: 53–55, 1996.

Stroescu, V. "The Experimental and Clinical Pharmacology of Procaine, Gerovital H3 and Aslavital." *Romanian Journal of Gerontology and Geriatrics*, 9:(4): 427–437, 1988.

Sullivan, K. "The evidence linking silver-mercury fillings to Alzheimer's disease: a literature review." *Townsend Letter for Doctors & Patients*, August/September, 1997.

Sunnen, G. "Ozone in medicine: overview and future direction." *Journal of Advancement in Medicine*, 1(3), 1988.

Suzuki, Y. "Alpha-lipoic acid is a potent inhibitor of NF-kB activation in human T cells." *Biochemical Biophysical Research Communication*, 189: 1709–1715, 1992.

Takagi, Y. "Calcium treatment of essential hypertension in elderly patients evaluated by 24 H monitoring." *American Journal of Hypertension*, 4: 836–839, 1991.

Takeuchi, T. "Pathology of Minamata disease." *Acta Pathology of Japan*, 32 (supplement 1): 73–99, 1982.

Tam, S. "Mesoprefrontal dopaminergic neurons: Can tyrosine availability influence their functions?" *Biochemical Pharmacology*, 53(4): 441–453, 1997.

Taussig, S. "The mechanism of the physiological action of bromelain." *Medical Hypothesis*, 29(1): 25–28, 1989.

Thienhaus, O. "A controlled double-blind study of high-dose dihydroergotoxine mesylate (Hydergine) in mild dementia." *Journal of American Geriatric Society*, 35(3): 219–223, March 1987.

Tollefson, G. "Short-term effects of the calcium channel blocker nimodipine (Bay-e-9736) in the management of primary degenerative dementia." *Biological Psychiatry,* 27(10): 1133–1142, 1990.

Trowbridge, J. *The Healing Powers of Chelation Therapy.* Stamford, CT: New Way of Life, Inc., 1992.

Turlapaty, P. "Magnesium deficiency produces spasms of coronary arteries: Relationship to etiology of sudden death ischemic heart disease." *Science,* 208: 199–200, 1980.

Valenzuela, A. "Silymarin protection against hepatic lipid peroxidation induced by acute ethanol intoxication in the rat." *Biological Pharmacology,* 34(12): 2209–2212, 1985.

Vernon, M. *Reversing Memory Loss.* Boston: Houghton Mifflin Company, 1992.

Vorhees, C. "Methamphetamine exposure during early postnatal development in rats." *Psychopharmacology,* 114(3): 392–401, 1994.

Wallace, L. "VOCs and the Environment and Public Health Exposure." H.J. Bloemen and J. Burn, editors, *Chemistry and Analysis of Volatile Organic Compounds in the Environment.* Glasgow, Scotland: Blackie Academic and Professional, 1993.

Wallin, A. "Blood-brain barrier function in vascular dementia." *ACTA, Neurological Scandanavia,* 81: 318–322, 1990.

Weiss, J. "Differential vulnerability to excitatory amino acid-induced toxicity and selective neuronal loss in neurodegenerative disease." *Canadian Journal of Neurological Science,* 18: 394–397, 1991.

Wilson, P. "Is coffee consumption a contributor to cardiovascular disease?" *Archives of Internal Medicine,* 149: 1169–1172, 1989.

Winocur, G. "A neuropsychological analysis of memory loss with age." *Neurobiology of Aging,* 9(5–6): 487–94, 1988.

Wong, P. "Ortho-substituted 2,2',3,5',6-Pentachlorobiphenyl (PCB 95) alters rat hippocampal ryanodine receptors and neuroplasticity in vitro: evidence for altered hippocampal functon." *Neuro Toxicology,* 18(2): 443–456, 1997.

Yamazaki, N. "Idebenone improves learning and memory impairment induced by cholinergic or serotonergic dysfunction in rats." *Archives of Gerontology and Geriatrics,* 8(3): 225–239, 1989.

Young, S. "Folic acid and psychopathology." *Progress in Neuropsychopharmacology and Biological Psychiatry*, 13: 841–863, 1989.

_____. "Some effects of dietary components (amino acids, carbohydrate, folic acid) on brain serotonin synthesis, mood, and behavior." *Canadian Journal of Physiology and Pharmacology*, 69: 893–903, 1989.

Index

A

ACAM. *See* American College of Advancement in Medicine.

Acetone, 89

Acetylcarnitine, supplementing with, 106–108

Acetylcholine, 29, 41, 48, 67

Acetylcholinesterase, 29

Acetyl-L-carnitine. *See* Acetylcarnitine.

Acquired immune deficiency syndrome (AIDS), 58

Adenosine triphosphate (ATP), 34, 35

Adrenaline, 23, 24, 45

AIDS. *See* Acquired immune deficiency syndrome.

Alcohol abuse, negative effects of, 50–51

Alexandra Avery Hair Oil, 82

Allergy elimination. *See* Nambudripad's Allergy Elimination Technique.

Alpha-lipoic acid, supplementing with, 109–110

Aluminum, 72, 84

Aluminum lakes, 82–83

Alzheimer's disease, 9, 14, 72, 75, 118, 136, 147, 152

Amalgam dental fillings, 74–75

American Board of Chelation Therapy, 168

American College of Advancement in Medicine (ACAM), 166–167, 168

American Dental Association, 74, 75

American ginseng. *See* Ginseng, supplementing with.

Amino acid, 65